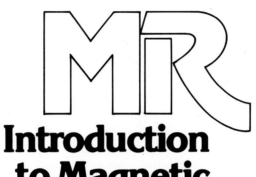

Introduction to Magnetic Resonance Imaging

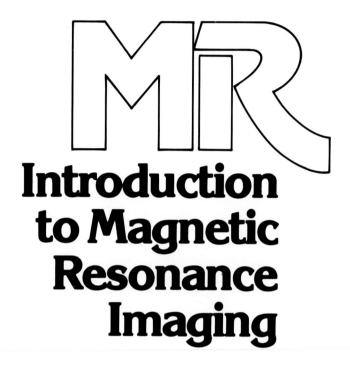

Introduction to Magnetic Resonance Imaging

Christopher J. Morgan, M.D.
William R. Hendee, Ph.D.

University of Colorado
School of Medicine
Denver, Colorado

The C.V. Mosby Co./Multi-Media Publishing, Inc.
St. Louis • Washington, D.C. • Toronto

© 1984 by Multi-Media Publishing, Inc.

First Edition

Printed in the United States of America

The C.V. Mosby Co./Multi-Media Publishing, Inc.
11830 Westline Industrial Drive
St. Louis, Missouri 63146

Library of Congress Cataloging in Publication Data

Hendee, William R.
  Introduction to magnetic resonance imaging.

  Includes bibliographical references and index.
  1. Nuclear magnetic resonance—Diagnostic use.
I. Morgan, Christopher J., 1950-   . II. Title.
III. Title: Introduction to magnetic resonance imaging.
[DNLM: 1. Diagnosis. 2. Nuclear Magnetic Resonance.
WB 141 H495i]
RC78.7.N83H46 1984   616.07'5   84-70467
ISBN 0-940122-13-8

MMP/M/M 9 8 7 6 5 4 3 2

To our wives Linda (C.J. Morgan) and
Jeannie (W.R. Hendee) for their support
and encouragement.

Special Acknowledgement
to Marvin L. Daves, M.D. in recognition
of sixteen years of stewardship
of the Department of Radiology
at the University of Colorado

Preface

The technology of nuclear magnetic resonance (NMR), and its applications to clinical medicine, have exploded over the past few years. Few would have predicted how far NMR would come in so short a time. In the imaging arena, how far it will go is impossible to forecast. There simply are too many unknowns, technical, clinical and financial. One characteristic is clear — NMR can produce exquisite images of patient anatomy in a variety of formats.

The principal potential applications of NMR to clinical medicine appear to be proton imaging and spectroscopic analysis of protons and other elements such as phosphorus and sodium. At the moment, only proton imaging is used clinically, and the closest competitor to NMR is computed tomography (CT). Since medicine is familiar with how CT works and what it does, since the initial applications of magnetic resonance imaging are in the central nervous system where CT has reigned supreme for over a decade, and since the price of a magnetic resonance imaging unit is equal to or somewhat greater than the cost of a CT scanner, NMR must be proven distinctly superior to CT if it is to become an important imaging modality. In many applications, NMR already has an edge over CT because of its improved contrast sensitivity and its ability to make sagittal, coronal and, ultimately, oblique sections directly.

The uniqueness of NMR in imaging lies partly in its sensitivity to blood flow, its ability to provide gated cardiac images, and its demonstration of changes in the relaxation parameters of tissues before there is obvious structural alteration. These capabilities suggest that NMR will be important in the diagnosis and management of a variety of cardiovascular conditions, central nervous system dysfunctions, metabolic abnormalities and tumors; institutions specializing in these areas that are considering the purchase of an additional CT scanner might well consider the acquisition of an NMR unit instead. Unfortunately, widespread clinical trials of NMR are only just beginning, and there are not yet enough data to recommend NMR to most hospitals. This observation is especially true in light of growing pressures to contain the costs of medical care. Few studies have yet been done to determine the cost effectiveness of NMR versus other modalities; this issue remains to be addressed in the near future.

Biochemical analysis of intact tissues by NMR was begun only a few years ago. So far, the results are exciting and have established a place for NMR as a tool for research into normal metabolism, metabolic disorders, and ischemia. The potential impact of spectroscopic NMR is great at the clinical level because of the sophisticated analysis it makes possible and because many of the more common diseases are relatively refractory to current treatments. It is conceivable that NMR ultimately will be able to define the portions of diseased tissue that are salvageable, to identify the best surgical or medical treatment, and to monitor its effectiveness. The latter is an area of great potential application of NMR.

Economic factors will largely determine how soon NMR becomes widely utilized as an imaging tool. The cost of a scanner (from $800,000 to $2.2 million) is high. Third-party reimbursement for NMR scans is not available at this time, and many hospitals currently cannot afford an NMR unit. By the time the reimbursement situation changes, much more will be known about the usefulness of NMR, primarily as a product of the experience gained from the use of scanners now being installed as experimental units in clinical sites. Hospitals will then be in a better position to decide whether they want an NMR unit and what type is best for them.

Nuclear magnetic resonance and its applications to medical imaging are technically complex topics. One of the major problems encountered by the individual interested in these topics, but lacking the appropriate physics and chemistry backgrounds, is the identification of interpretable sources of information. The production of such a source was our principal intent in the preparation of this text.

In the clinical arena, some aversion has surfaced in the use of the term **nuclear** in conjunction with magnetic resonance. As a consequence, the expression **magnetic resonance imaging** is gaining popularity as a description of the imaging applications of nuclear magnetic resonance. In this text, magnetic resonance (MR) will be used in the context of imaging applications; non-imaging applications (e.g., spectroscopy) will be referenced as nuclear magnetic resonance (NMR).

Persons with widely disparate backgrounds are being drawn into the culture of magnetic resonance imaging. Physicians specializing in medical imaging, as well as many others who foresee useful applications of nuclear magnetic resonance for their patients, are a potential audience for this book. Physicists and engineers with solid technical backgrounds but without detailed knowledge of MR and its clinical applications hopefully will find the text helpful. Technologists who ultimately will be the operators of MR imaging units are another group of potential readers. For all of these individuals, and to others who have a need for a text of this type, we hope that the book satisfies their requirements.

In preparing the text, we have learned from and leaned upon many who have preceded us in their involvement in nuclear magnetic resonance. Nevertheless, any errors and misconceptions remain our own responsibility; we hope they are few in number and severity.

Finally, we are indebted to colleagues too numerous to mention who supported this effort, corrected our mistakes, and encouraged the completion of the text when interruptions pulled us away. We especially appreciate the patience of Ms. Rita Taylor in typing numerous redrafts as we attempted to keep the text current over its period of production. Of particular significance are the many contributions of our administrative assistant, Ms. Linda Taylor. How she managed to keep the text in order in the presence of our chaotic working habits remains a mystery to both of us.

Christopher J. Morgan, M.D.
William R. Hendee, Ph.D.

Table of Contents

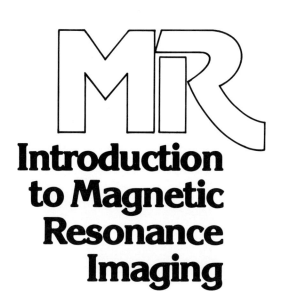

Introduction
to Magnetic
Resonance
Imaging

Chapter 1
The Evolution of Nuclear Magnetic Resonance

The origin of nuclear magnetic resonance (NMR) can be traced to efforts at the turn of the century to explain the wavelengths of visible light and ultraviolet radiation emitted by various substances. Spectroscopy using visible and ultraviolet light had been developed in the late 1800s and was useful in detecting the presence of certain elements in unknown compounds. However, not all of the observed light patterns could be explained. This mystery occupied the efforts of a number of physicists who proposed various models to explain the structure of the atom and the way electrons interacted with each other and with the nucleus inside the atom. Even more mysterious was the observation that each wavelength of emitted light split into two wavelengths when a substance was placed in a magnetic field. It was not until 1924 that Pauli realized that the splitting was caused by magnetic interactions between the nucleus and electrons, and that these interactions were affected by an external magnetic field. These explanations correlated well with experimental data; however, it meant that the nucleus must have magnetic properties.

For the next few years, many physicists became preoccupied with measurements of the magnetic properties of nuclei, especially those of hydrogen since it is the simplest element (ordinary hydrogen has one proton and no neutrons in the nucleus). In 1933, Stern and his colleagues investigated the deflection of a beam of H_2 molecules in a nonhomogeneous magnetic field (1, 2). They observed that the beam split into components that followed slightly different paths as a result of interaction between the magnetic field and the magnetic properties of the protons. By measuring the deflection, they arrived at an estimate of the magnetic moment of the proton that was accurate to within a small percentage. The same investigators later performed a similar experiment with deuterium, an isotope of hydrogen with a proton and a single neutron in its nucleus. These experiments revealed that the neutron also has a magnetic moment. This result was unexpected because the neutron has no net electrical charge.

A decisive step in understanding the magnetic properties of nuclei was achieved when Rabi, one of Stern's former students, designed an apparatus that furnished two regions of a strong, uniform magnetic field that were separated by an alternating magnetic field oscillating in the radiofrequency (rf) range (**Figure 1-1**). The static magnetic field at one end of the apparatus was of equal intensity but opposite orientation to the field at the other end. For all molecules traversing the apparatus without influence from the rf field, the path in the first static field was exactly compensated by the path in the opposite static field at the far end of the apparatus. Hence, these molecules would be detected on the centerline of the apparatus. On the other hand, if the magnetic moment of a molecule changed in orientation as it passed through the rf field, the second static field would no longer exactly compensate for the first and the molecule would arrive at the detector in a location off the centerline of the apparatus. This behavior of a molecule in an rf-alternating magnetic field of prescribed frequency is the principle of nuclear magnetic resonance.

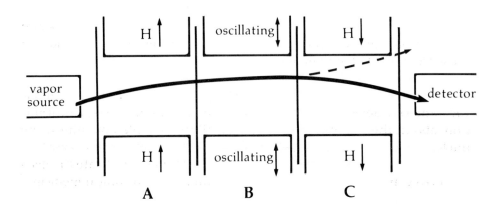

Figure 1-1. The Rabi apparatus. Regions **A** and **C** have strong magnetic fields but the orientation of the field in **C** is opposite to that in **A**. Region **B** has a magnetic field oscillating at a radiofrequency that can be varied experimentally. Molecules unaffected in region **B** are deflected in equal but opposite ways in regions **A** and **C** and emerge from the apparatus with no net deflection. If the frequency of the oscillating field in region **B** is set equal to the Larmor frequency of the nuclei of interest in the molecules, the orientation of some nuclei will change and they will be deflected away from the centerline (dotted line) in region **C**. These molecules will be detected only when the detector is moved off-center.

In practice, the rf field of the Rabi apparatus was varied until a maximum deflection from centerline was observed for the molecules arriving at the end of the apparatus. From knowledge of the frequency for maximum deflection, nuclear magnetic moments could be computed with an accuracy exceeding 99%. Rabi's first experiments in 1938 were with LiCl molecules (3). Later experiments with deuterium and hydrogen-deuterium molecules led to the detection of asymmetrical forces between the proton and neutron that confirmed the suspicion that the distribution of charge in nuclear particles is asymmetric (4). This finding supported the hypothesis that the proton and neutron may not be fundamental particles. In 1944, Rabi received a Nobel prize for his work.

Rabi's work represents a fundamental breakthrough in understanding the magnetic properties of nuclei. Yet, his apparatus suffered from two fundamental limitations. The first was that only substances that existed naturally as gases, or that could be vaporized, were subject to examination because they had to traverse the entire length of the apparatus. Second, measurement of the deflection of a molecular beam is a rather indirect way of demonstrating nuclear magnetic resonance. These limitations were overcome in 1945 in similar experiments performed independently by Bloch (5) and Purcell (6). They were able to measure the magnetic properties of the proton to within one part per million, an accuracy that exceeded the scope of the prevailing theory of nuclear forces. Bloch and Purcell were awarded a Nobel prize in 1952.

Bloch and Purcell recognized that certain nuclei will resonate and emit a radio signal if they are placed in a strong magnetic field and pulsed with radiofrequency energy. Efforts by these investigators to detect the very weak radio signal were successful and established the foundation for all the work on NMR to follow. Analysis of the amplitude and frequency distributions of the emitted signal yields information about the chemical composition of the sample containing the nuclei. This analysis is the principle of NMR spectroscopy, an analytic technique of considerable value, initially in chemistry, later in biochemistry and animal physiology, and potentially in clinical medicine.

Researchers used Bloch's and Purcell's methods to study nuclear magnetic resonance in a variety of ways. For example, minute differences could be expected in the resonance frequency of a nucleus within a chemical compound because electrons in atoms near the nucleus would shield the nucleus to varying degrees. Experiments to detect these minute frequency shifts required a homogeneous magnetic field to 1 part in 10^8 so that the inhomogeneity of the magnetic field caused by the electron cloud around the nucleus would not be overshadowed by magnetic field inhomogeneities attributable to the equipment. By the late 1940s, a variety of research groups had produced satisfactory magnetic fields and had demonstrated frequency shifts for nuclei such as phosphorus-31, fluorine-19, and nitrogen-15. It was immediately recognized that analysis of the "chemical shift" could help chemists deduce the structure of chemical compounds. Further progress in magnet technology in Bloch's laboratory at Stanford in 1951 led to identification of chemical shifts of protons in the first biologically important compound, ethanol. These results stimulated the finding that simple frequency shifts in organic chemical groups could be used to delineate the chemical structure of organic compounds by NMR techniques.

For the past three decades, NMR in chemistry has been characterized by expansion into a variety of subfields, with a wealth of additional applications. At first, much of the work was on applied problems such as NMR studies of polymers, coal, and the water content of agricultural materials. Later refinements permitted chemists to measure the rates at which chemical groups are exchanged among molecules. These measurements led to the development of high-resolution spectroscopy and made it possible to examine biological materials and crystalline solids. The field of NMR spectroscopy has grown so fast that there are now six review series, four journals, and over 5,000 articles per year devoted to the chemical applications of NMR. In the words of Packard (7): "Chemists got the point very quickly, thanked the physicists and took over."

There are three principal reasons for the outstanding success of NMR in chemistry. First, it is relatively straightforward to interpret spectra in terms of fundamental properties of chemical compounds so that a large amount of information can be extracted from experiments. Second, new discoveries have given continued vitality to the field. Third, remarkable progress has been made in instrumentation and analytical techniques.

One technical development was especially important. The original experimental technique involved measurement of the absorption of energy by a sample while the frequency of the oscillating magnetic field was slowly varied (or conversely, while the intensity of the static magnetic field was slowly varied at a fixed radiofrequency). This approach is relatively slow and inefficient because it measures the absorption by the sample one frequency at a time. The modern technique of pulse NMR was proposed by Hahn in 1950 (8). In this method, the sample is exposed to a pulse of radiofrequency energy containing a range of frequencies. This approach had relatively few applications until 1957, when it was noted that Fourier transformation (FT) of the signal emitted by the sample produces a spectrum equivalent to that obtained by the absorption method. A Fourier transformation is a mathematical technique to separate a signal into distinct frequencies. With the FT method, the NMR spectrum can be gathered much more quickly simply by repeating the pulse series a number of times and summing the data prior to Fourier transformation. Widespread use of pulse NMR techniques was delayed a few years until advances in solid state electronics and computer technology made it feasible to include FT capabilities in NMR spectrometers used for routine work. Today, almost all spectrometers and NMR imaging units are pulse FT systems.

The full application of NMR to the study of biological systems did not occur until the mid-1960s because the spectroscopy of carbon requires FT techniques, signal summation by computer, and high-strength superconducting magnets. Subsequent applications include analyses of the structure and interactions of nucleic acids and proteins in solution, and studies of internal protein structure, the conformation of enzymes, and metabolic pathways in living cells.

The application of NMR to clinical medicine originated at the State University of New York campus in Brooklyn, where Damadian was investigating the relaxation behavior of water in bacterial cells as a function of the intracellular concentration of sodium and potassium (9). Since it had been shown previously (10) that the balance of alkali ions may be altered in cancer, Damadian extended his studies to examination of the relaxation characteristics of tumors. He found that the relaxation constants of certain tumors in rats were prolonged compared to normal tissues, and suggested that these constants might permit discrimination of cancerous from normal tissue (11). He subsequently extended his work to humans (12) and suggested that NMR relaxation measurements in the operating room could help identify the malignancy of excised tissues, thus supplementing pathological examination. He also patented an NMR device designed to detect and localize cancer in the body by means of its abnormal relaxation behavior. Although subsequent work has shown that the distinction between normal and cancerous tissue on the basis of relaxation parameters is more difficult than originally postulated by Damadian, these first results were exciting and attracted international attention.

At the State University of New York in Stony Brook, Lauterbur began to explore the possibility of producing images by NMR techniques. In 1973, (13) he proposed an imaging method he termed zeugmatography (from the Greek **zeugma**, "that which joins together"). This method is based on computer reconstruction of an image from projections, a method used in x-ray transmission computed tomography. The first MR image was reconstructed from four projections through two water-filled capillary tubes. The rather crude image was the beginning of all MR imaging techniques in use today.

NMR signals are very weak and subject to noise interference from a variety of sources. This problem has been addressed in the chemistry laboratory by extending NMR observations over several hours and using a computer to average the results of thousands of individual pulse experiments. In the clinical setting, however, many patients per day must be examined and rapid imaging is a necessity. Also, prolonged scanning times yield images degraded by patient motion. In most instances, a chemical sample is homogeneous and only a small portion needs to be evaluated; on the other hand, every point in the head, thorax, or abdomen must be sampled for magnetic resonance imaging. The need to obtain a strong signal and to sample a large number of points meant that totally new equipment had to be designed for magnetic resonance imaging. Many technical problems had to be overcome, and funding was limited because it was unknown whether NMR would ever produce clinically useful images.

Magnetic resonance imaging (MR) equipment has many components including wires, coils, magnets, amplifiers, and other complex circuit elements. The parts that generate the radiofrequencies and magnetic field gradients must deliver high-intensity electrical currents and switch them on and off rapidly with precise timing. Performance of the antennas and receiving circuits must be optimized, and high-gain, low-noise amplifiers are required. Magnets must be built that produce strong fields with a nonuniformity of less than one part in a hundred thousand over a large volume. The system components interact with each other and are also influenced by both the patient and the environment. Design of a satisfactory MR system was a challenging proposition, and there were those who thought it could not be done.

The MR signal from a specimen may be sampled point by point, or simultaneously from all the points in a line, plane, or entire volume. Since all points in the specimen must eventually be sampled, and since the signal is easier to detect when more points are sampled at the same time, it was soon realized that the best imaging methods are (theoretically) those which sample an entire plane or volume at once. As the number of sampled points increases, however, so does the complexity of the applied magnetic field gradients and the data storage and processing requirements. Planar and volumetric methods of data sampling have been achieved only in the last few years.

The first imaging experiments were performed with the slower continuous wave methods used originally in spectroscopy. Fourier transformation techniques for imaging were first proposed by Kumar et al. in 1975 (14). These techniques have the advantage that an image can be reconstructed by straightforward computer techniques, and image quality is less dependent on the quality of the magnetic field. Their disadvantage is that some of the signal is lost during each imaging cycle as the additional magnetic gradients required by FT methods are applied. This loss can be minimized by using very strong magnetic gradients; however, strong gradients place a greater demand on the equipment.

The first image of a biological specimen (a mouse) was obtained in 1974 at the University of Aberdeen, Scotland (15). Twenty-five projections obtained over a one-hour imaging time were used to generate T_1 relaxation data, which were then ranked on a 10-point color-coded scale. (T_1 and T_2 relaxation constants are explained in detail in Chapter 2). Approximately 1,200 such points were printed out by computer and colored in by hand. Not only were the mouse's major organs visible, but the darkest area in the image, corresponding to the longest relaxation time, represented edema around a neck fracture. Demonstration of this pathology encouraged the Aberdeen group to order a magnet specifically for human imaging. The magnet was delivered in 1977.

In the meantime Damadian, using a method called field focusing NMR (FONAR), published images of a live rat with an implanted tumor (16) and of a human chest (17). In its earlier stages, the FONAR technique sampled the tissue region one point at a time. At about the same time, researchers at the University of Nottingham, England, devised a line scan method in which all the points along a line were sampled simultaneously. A planar image was compiled by moving the line incrementally through the specimen (18). Scan times were reduced significantly compared to the original FONAR method because the whole line could be examined in about the same time as a single point. The results were encouraging enough to order a system large enough to examine the human torso.

In 1978, the first line scan images of a human abdomen were obtained (19). These images permitted only dim recognition of major organs and blood vessels. The particular line scan technique used for these images yielded a complicated MR signal that was difficult to analyze and that caused a loss of resolution. This difficulty was an inherent problem in the technique and was never resolved.

The Aberdeen group developed an improved line scan method and demonstrated human images that were improved over those from Nottingham. However, these images were degraded by motion artifacts that arose because the image was formed by subtracting two signals obtained at slightly different times (20). Workers at Aberdeen realized that their magnet did not generate a sufficiently uniform magnetic field for projection reconstruction, and worked unsuccessfully on adapting the original two-dimensional FT technique to their experiments. Eventually the reconstruction problem was overcome by applying radiofrequency pulses of constant duration but different amplitudes, rather than pulses of constant amplitude but different durations, as suggested in the original FT paper. This minor change improved system performance significantly, and the Aberdeen "spin warp" method began to furnish good images in 1980 (21), leading to a series of clinical trials that are still being conducted.

Another research group at Nottingham produced images of the wrist and forearm (22) by a different line scan technique. Alternating perpendicular magnetic gradients were used to select a line in the specimen; this line was moved sequentially through the specimen to obtain an image. The use of alternating gradients simplified the imaging procedure and solved some of the resolution problems of other line scan methods. Image resolution was improved and bones, muscle, tendons, and arteries were clearly demonstrated. The authors were encouraged to expand their method to planar scanning by using a single time-varying magnetic gradient. In 1980, this Nottingham group produced the first successful image of the brain (23). (The team disbanded after several of its members accepted positions in the United States.)

Scientists at EMI Ltd. in England became interested in the work at Aberdeen and other sites and built an imaging unit with the help of consultants from Nottingham. They produced their first image of the head in 1977 with a resistive magnet, using projection reconstruction. In 1979, EMI Ltd. joined with Hammersmith Hospital in England to build a superconducting magnet system. From data already published, the group felt that various normal and abnormal tissues could be discriminated on the basis of the relaxation constants T_1 and T_2. They chose both T_1-weighted and T_2-weighted imaging methods and obtained excellent results. The methods of data acquisition developed by the EMI-Hammersmith coalition are still widely used in MR imaging.

In 1981, the first published results of the EMI-Hammersmith team revealed high-quality brain images (24). This work was followed shortly by the first major clinical trial of MR imaging. Subsequently, the original projection reconstruction method was changed to a two-dimensional FT technique with simultaneous acquisition of multiple images, resulting in excellent images with significantly reduced imaging times and less image degradation caused by patient motion.

Another stage in the development of a clinical imaging system began on the campus of the University of California at San Francisco (UCSF). Technical problems were circumvented at first by the use of a line scan method designed to avoid motion artifacts. The lines were defined by a selective excitation process developed at UCSF (25), and FT techniques were used. Early results with animals in a 30-cm. bore magnet system were successful, and a superconducting unit designed for patient studies was constructed. The data acquisition process was expanded to a planar method, and the important capability of image acquisition from multiple planes in one imaging period was added (26). With this approach, the time spent waiting between repetitive image sequences while the magnetization relaxes in a particular imaging plane can be used to collect data from other imaging planes. The "multi-slice" technique overcomes many of the difficult data handling problems encountered with three-dimensional volumetric methods of data acquisition. At the same time it reduces imaging times significantly compared to those for single plane techniques.

None of the imaging systems described above utilizes a magnetic field that is strong or homogeneous enough to permit NMR spectroscopy. Initially it was widely believed that imaging would not be possible with a system capable of spectroscopy, because the intense magnetic field required for spectroscopy would yield signals of frequencies too high to penetrate the tissues of interest. This was disproven in 1982 when high field images and phosphorus spectra of the brain were demonstrated (27). This success sparked the hope that both imaging and chemical analysis will someday be part of a routine MR examination. Currently, it is not possible to do both simultaneously, and the clinical value of chemical analysis by MR has yet to be proven.

At the moment, there are several areas of MR imaging research, all of which are concerned with maximizing image contrast and decreasing imaging time without loss of resolution. Most manufacturers are investigating imaging applications in the 0.15 to 1.5 tesla range of magnetic field strengths, and various claims and counterclaims are being made about the optimum magnetic field strength for proton imaging and for spectroscopy. Manufacturers and other investigators are refining pulse techniques to maximize tissue contrast and minimize artifacts. Three-dimensional FT techniques have yet to be perfected. Some investigators have demonstrated gated acquisition of data for cardiac studies, and others are pursuing flow measurements by MR techniques. Contrast agents for MR are being investigated, and many researchers are exploring the correlation between relaxation characteristics and the fundamental properties of tissues.

References

1. Friesch, R., and Stern, O.: Uber die magnetische ablenkung von wasserstoff — Molekulen und das magnetische moment das protons I. Z. Physik 85:4-16, 1933.

2. Esterman, I., and Stern, O.: Uber die magnetische ablenkung von wasserstoff — Molekulen und das magnetische moment das protons II. Z. Physik 85:17-24, 1933.

3. Rabi, I.I., and others: Molecular beam resonance method for measuring nuclear magnetic moments. Phys. Rev. 55:526-535, 1939.

4. Kellogg, J.M.B., Rabi, I.I., and Ramsey, N.F.: An electrical quadrapole moment of the deutron. The radiofrequency spectra of HD and D_2 molecules in a magnetic field. Phys. Rev. 57:677-695, 1940.

5. Bloch, F.: The principle of nuclear induction. In *Nobel Lectures in Physics: 1946-1962.* New York: 1964, Elsevier Publishing Company.

6. Purcell, E.M.: Research in nuclear magnetism. In *Nobel Lectures in Physics: 1946-1962.* New York: 1964, Elsevier Publishing Company.

7. Rogers, E., Packard, E.M., and Shoolery, J.N.: *The Origins of NMR Spectroscopy.* Palo Alto, CA, 1963: Varian Associates.

8. Hahn, E.L.: Spin echoes. Phys. Rev. 80:580-594, 1950.

9. Damadian, R.: Biological ion exchanger resins. I: Quantitative electrostatic correspondence of fixed charge and mobile counter ion. Biophys. J. 11:739-760, 1971.

10. Ling, G.N.: *A Physical Theory of the Living State.* Waltham, MA: 1962, Blaisdell.

11. Damadian, R.: Tumor detection by nuclear magnetic resonance. Science 171:1151-1153, 1971.

12. Damadian, R., and others: Nuclear magnetic resonance as a new tool in cancer research: Human tumors by NMR. Ann. NY Acad. Sci. 222:1048-1076, 1973.

13. Lauterbur, P.C.: Image formation by induced local interactions: Examples employing nuclear magnetic resonance. Nature (London) 242:190-191, 1973.

14. Kumar, A., Welti, I., and Ernst R.R.: NMR Fourier zeugmatography. J. Mag. Reson. 18:69-83, 1975.

15. Mallard, J., and others: Imaging by nuclear magnetic resonance and its bio-medical implications. J. Biomed. Eng. 1:153-160, 1979.

16. Damadian, R., and others: Field focusing nuclear magnetic resonance (FONAR): Visualization of a tumor in a live animal. Science 194:1430-1431, 1976.

17. Damadian, R., Goldsmith, M., and Minkoff, L.: NMR in cancer: XVI. FONAR image of the live human body. Physiol. Chem. Phys. 9:97-100, 1977.

18. Mansfield, P., and Maudsley, A.A.: Medical imaging by NMR. Brit. J. Radiol. 50:188-194, 1977.

19. Mansfield, P., and others: Short Communications — human whole body line-scan imaging by NMR. Brit. J. Radiol. 51:921-922, 1978.

20. Mallard, J., and others: *In vivo* N.M.R. imaging in medicine. The Aberdeen approach, both physical and biological. Phil. Trans. R. Soc. Land. 289:519-533, 1980.

21. Edelstein, W.A., and others: Spin warp NMR imaging and applications to human whole-body imaging. Phys. Med. Biol. 25:751-756, 1980.

22. Hinshaw, W.S., Bottomley, P.A., and Holland, G.N.: Radiographic thin-section image of the human wrist by nuclear magnetic resonance. Nature (London) 270:722-723, 1977.

23. Holland, G.N., Moore, W.S., and Hawkes, R.C.: Nuclear magnetic resonance tomography of the brain. J. Comp. Assist. Tomog. 4:1-3, 1980.

24. Doyle, F.H., and others: Imaging of the brain by nuclear magnetic resonance. Lancet 2:53-57, 1981.

25. Crooks, L.E.: Selective irradiation line scan techniques for NMR imaging. IEEE Trans. Nuc. Sci. 3:1239-1241, 1980.

26. Crooks, L.E., and others: Nuclear magnetic resonance whole body imager operating at 3.5 KGauss. Radiology 143:169-174, 1982.

27. Bottomley, P.A., and others: Anatomy and metabolism of the normal brain studied by magnetic resonance at 1.5 Tesla. Radiology 150:441-446, 1984.

Chapter 2
Physical Principles of Magnetic Resonance Imaging

Obtaining A Magnetic Resonance Signal

Electrons, protons, and neutrons are all elementary particles whose basic properties have been understood for many years. Electrons carry a minute negative charge and protons have a positive charge of the same magnitude. Neutrons have no net charge. All three particles possess a property called **spin**, and may be thought of as spinning rapidly on their own axes like tiny tops. The combination of spin and electric charge produces a small circulating current in each particle that results in the creation of a tiny magnetic field around the particle. Although neutrons have no net electric charge, they appear to have a charge distribution that is somewhat asymmetrical. This non-uniform distribution of charge and the spin of the neutron means that it also has a tiny magnetic field.

In the nucleus, each neutron and proton spins on its axis, yielding a magnetic moment that causes the particle to behave like a small magnet. In most nuclei, the neutrons and protons align so that their spins and magnetizations cancel. Complete cancellation is not possible, however, if the number of protons or neutrons is odd. In hydrogen, for example, the nucleus contains a solitary proton. This proton generates a small magnetic field, represented by a vector along the axis of spin. In a substance with nuclei containing one or more unpaired protons or neutrons (e.g., hydrogen-1; carbon-13; fluorine-19; sodium-23 and phosphorus-31), the nuclei are oriented randomly so that the substance possesses no net magnetization. When a magnetic field is applied to the substance, however, many of the nuclei become oriented either parallel or antiparallel to the magnetic field (**Figure 2-1**). Usually there are considerably more nuclei oriented parallel than antiparallel to the applied field. The nuclei in the two orientations differ in energy; however, the energy difference is very slight (about 1/1000 of thermal energy at body temperature). The energy difference, as well as the number of nuclei oriented antiparallel to the applied field, increases with the strength of the applied magnetic field. Once nuclei have been aligned in this fashion, the distribution of nuclei between the two energy states can be altered by applying a small pulse of radiofrequency energy to the substance.

13

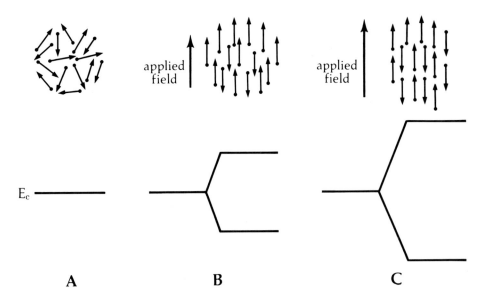

Figure 2-1. A, energy levels for protons in the absence of a magnetic field. **B,** the presence of a magnetic field. **C,** the presence of a stronger magnetic field where the energy separation is greater.

The orientation of the nuclei induces a net magnetization, termed the magnetic moment, in the sample. With such a magnetized sample, application of a small low-energy pulse of the proper frequency will cause the sample to absorb some of the energy. In response, the sample's magnetic moment will tilt out of alignment with the applied magnetic field. In the tilted orientation, the magnetic moment begins a motion called precession, in which it rotates slowly in a path that describes the wall of a cone (**Figure 2-2**). The frequency of rotation (i.e., the precessional frequency) varies with the sample and the strength of the applied field. The rotation causes the emission of a radiofrequency (rf) signal from the sample (**Figure 2-3**). The frequency of this signal is identical to the precessional frequency and is termed the Larmor frequency (ω). The Larmor frequency is the product of the magnetic field strength (β) and the gyromagnetic ratio (γ) of the nuclei in the sample:

$$\omega = \gamma\beta$$

where the gyromagnetic ratio is the ratio of the magnetic moment of the nuclei to their angular momentum.

The Larmor frequency is unique for each type of nucleus; in a given magnetic field, therefore, all identical nuclei (e.g., hydrogen nuclei in similar molecular configurations) emit a signal of the same frequency. The frequency of this signal varies only with the magnetic field strength. This feature is important in encoding the signal with spatial information in the process of forming a magnetic resonance image.

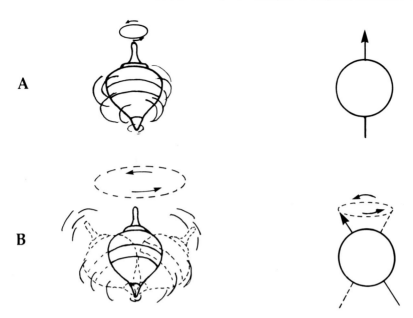

A

B

Figure 2-2. The motion of precession. A, a child's top and a magnetic moment oriented by a magnetic field will both maintain their orientation if undisturbed. **B**, when they are bumped off-axis by a finger or a radiofrequency pulse of energy, respectively, they begin a new rotational motion called precession.

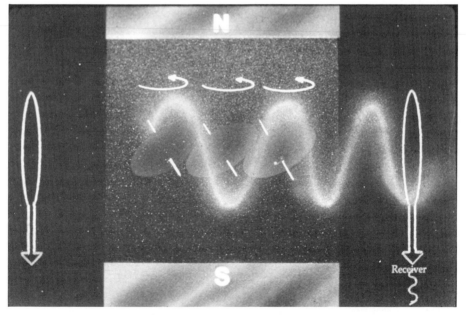

Figure 2-3. As the magnetic moment of a sample precesses about the direction of the applied magnetic field, radiofrequency energy is radiated at the Larmor frequency.

Decay of the Magnetic Resonance Signal

After the magnetic moment of a sample is pulsed out of alignment with the applied field, it tends gradually to become realigned with the field. The realignment process occurs as nuclei return to a lower energy state by releasing energy to the lattice of atoms around the nuclei. This form of realignment is termed spin-lattice relaxation. (Relaxation is any process whereby a system returns to its original state after absorbing energy.) At the same time, the precessing magnetic moment tends to separate into components (e.g., break apart) through a dephasing process termed spin-spin relaxation. Both relaxation processes contribute to decay of the radiofrequency signal emitted from the sample. It is important to understand these processes because they determine the appearance of various tissues in a magnetic resonance image.

Relaxation processes can be explained simply by a conceptual scheme called the rotating frame of reference in which precession is represented by a single stationary vector in the zy plane of a three-dimensional coordinate system (**Figure 2-4**). The central angle of the cone of precession (θ) corresponds to the angle between the magnetization vector and the applied magnetic field.

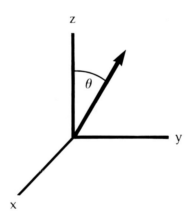

Figure 2-4. Rotating frame of reference, with precession represented by a single stationary vector.

Spin-lattice relaxation involves the gradual return of the magnetic moment of a sample into alignment with the applied magnetic field. As the angle θ decreases, the intensity of the emitted radio signal decreases (**Figure 2-5**), until eventually the sample's magnetic moment is once again aligned with the applied field. The rate at which the magnetic moment (M) realigns with the applied field over time (t) is described mathematically as:

$$M = M_o \ (1 - e^{-t/T_1})$$

16

in which T_1 is the spin-lattice relaxation time and M_o is the original magnetization aligned with the applied field. Different substances have different T_1 values, signifying that spin-lattice relaxation occurs at different rates in different substances because of differences in the interaction between the precessing magnetic moment and the particular molecular lattice. The signal in a substance with short T_1 decays faster than that from a substance with long T_1. Representative T_1 values for various tissue constitutents are shown in Table 1. These values are appropriate for magnetic field strengths of 0.2 tesla; in higher fields, the T_1 values are somewhat greater because the efficiency of the relaxation process is diminished.

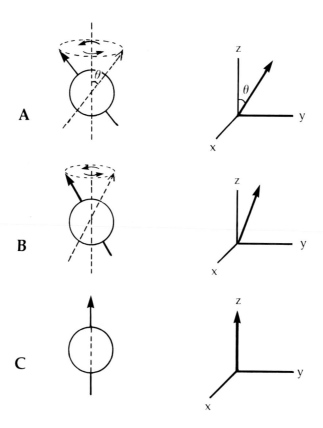

Figure 2-5. Spin-lattice relaxation diagrammed in the rotating frame of reference. A, the precession of the magnetic moment of a sample is represented by a cone swept out by the magnetization vector in a standard coordinate system, or by a single, stationary vector at an angle θ with the applied field in a rotating frame of reference. **B,** as the magnetic moment reorients toward the applied field by spin-lattice relaxation (T_1), θ decreases. **C,** eventually, the magnetic moment of the sample once again lies along the z axis in the direction of the applied field. (Reprinted with permission from the Western Journal of Medicine. In press.)

Table 1*

T_1 and T_2 values in msec for normal tissues and for pathological specimens at 0.2T. Values are reported as mean values and standard deviations.

Tissue	T_1		T_2	
fat	240 ±	20	60 ±	10
muscle	400 ±	40	50 ±	10
liver	380 ±	20	40 ±	20
pancreas	290 ±	20	60 ±	40
spleen	420 ±	50	20	
kidney	670 ±	60	50 ±	10
parotid gland	350		30	
arteries (aorta)	860 ±	510	90 ±	50
bone marrow (vertebra)	380 ±	50	70 ±	20
bone marrow (long bones)	280 ±	40	80 ±	10
bile	890 ±	140	80 ±	20
urine	2,200 ±	610	570 ±	230
pleural effusion	2,200 ±	1,930	300 ±	20
liver metastases	570 ±	190	40 ±	10
liver abscess	1,180		100	
pancreatic carcinoma	840		40	
pancreatic pseudocyst	1,130		70	
pancreatitis	300		150	
adrenal carcinoma	570 ±	160	110 ±	40
parotid gland sarcoma	620		40	
lung carcinoma	940 ±	460	20 ±	10
lung atelectasis	720		110	
prostatic carcinoma	610 ±	60	140 ±	90
bladder carcinoma	660 ±	280	140 ±	110
lymphoma (abdominal)	650 ±	200	110 ±	70
breast carcinoma	460		180	
osteomyelitis	770 ±	20	220 ±	40
bone necrosis (hip)	1,240		60	
bone metastasis (osteoblastic)	390		220	

*(Reprinted with permission from N. Rupp, M. Reiser, E. Stetter, The Diagnostic Value of Morphology and Relaxation Times in NMR-Imaging of the Body, Europ. J. Radiol. 3, 68-76, 1983.)

Spin-spin relaxation occurs by a different mechanism. The precession of the tilted magnetic moment is influenced by small inhomogeneities in the surrounding magnetic field and by interaction of individual nuclei one with another. These processes cause the precessing magnetic moment to separate or dephase into components, leading to a loss in signal intensity. This dephasing process is termed spin-spin relaxation T_2. (Phase describes a state of synchrony among different events; events are said to "dephase" or "go out of phase" when the synchronization diminishes.)

Spin-spin relaxation in a rotating reference frame is depicted in **Figure 2-6**: In **A**, the magnetic moment of the sample is aligned with the

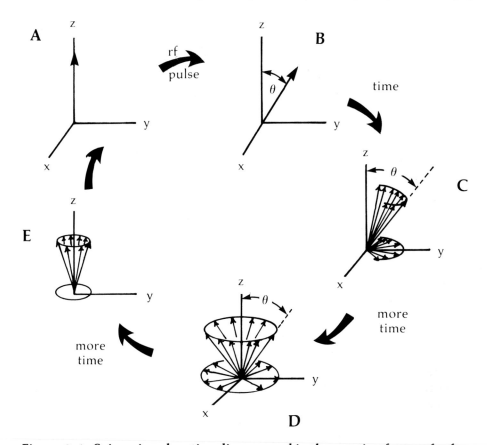

Figure 2-6. Spin-spin relaxation diagrammed in the rotating frame of reference. A, the magnetic moment of the sample is aligned with the magnetic field. **B**, immediately following an rf pulse, the magnetic moment of the sample can be represented by a single vector. **C**, as the magnetization vector begins to break up or dephase due to localized nonuniformities in the applied field, components of the vector begin to fan out in the xy plane. **D**, when there are an equal number of components in all directions in the xy plane, the components cancel one another and the MR signal disappears. **E**, as time passes, the cone representing the precessing but dephased magnetic moment continues to narrow because of spin-lattice relaxation. **A**, finally, the magnetic moment once again is realigned with the applied field. (Reprinted with permission from the Western Journal of Medicine. In press.)

applied magnetic field; in **B**, the magnetic moment is tilted out of alignment by an rf pulse, and the magnetic moment begins to precess about the applied field; in **C**, localized inhomogeneities in the applied field and spin-spin interactions among nuclei cause the precessing magnetic moment to separate into various components that precess at slightly different rates. This dephasing process, termed spin-spin relaxation T_2, leads to a decay in signal intensity characterized by the expression:

$$M = M_o (1-e^{-t/T_2})$$

When the dephasing process is complete (**Figure 2-6, D**), each xy component of the signal is balanced by a component in the opposite direction, and the signal intensity falls to zero. Still, the magnetization vector continues to realign with the applied field (**Figure 2-6, E**) until realignment is complete (**Figure 2-6, A**). Representative T_2 values for various tissue constituents at 0.2T are shown in Table 1.

Spin-spin relaxation and spin-lattice relaxation are separate processes caused by different interactive mechanisms. Variations in molecular structure or chemical composition produce changes in the rates of each type of relaxation, reflected by differences in T_1 and T_2. The only generalization possible is that T_2 can approach but never exceed T_1.

Variations in Relaxation Constants

Three variables influence the strength of the proton magnetic resonance signal. These variables are the concentration of protons and the relaxation constants T_1 and T_2. In most tissues, the concentration of protons is related principally to the water content and secondarily to the lipid content. Images that reflect only proton density (also called "spin density") do not yield as much tissue contrast as do images that also reflect T_1 and T_2. The maximum contrast available with spin density images is less because the range of variation in spin density is only about 30%; variations in T_1 and T_2 are significantly greater. In routine spin density images of the brain, for example, the contrast between gray and white matter is comparable to that in CT images (**Figure 2-7**).

Spin-lattice relaxation occurs with the help of thermal motion in the sample. As thermal motion increases, energy transfer processes also increase and relaxation by spin-lattice interactions occurs more readily. Since temperature is a measure of thermal motion, increasing the temperature of a sample leads to a reduction in T_1.

T_1 varies from one tissue to another (Table 1). In solids, the atoms are held rigidly in place by interatomic bonds and they rarely collide with each other. This rigidity leads to relatively long spin-lattice relaxation times, with T_1 values often on the order of many seconds or more. Most biological tissues are more liquid-like in their T_1 behavior; for example, most water in tissue is in a relatively unbound condition and the molecules move and collide frequently. These molecules provide "thermal contact" in the interstices of tissues and accelerate the process of spin-lattice relaxation. Hence, T_1 values for most soft tissues are measured in msec (e.g., typical brain parenchyma T_1s are about 700 msec at magnetic field strengths of 0.3-0.5T).

Spin-spin relaxation T_2 depends upon the interaction of the magnetization vector with localized nonuniformities in the applied field as well as interactions among individual nuclei in the sample. In a solid,

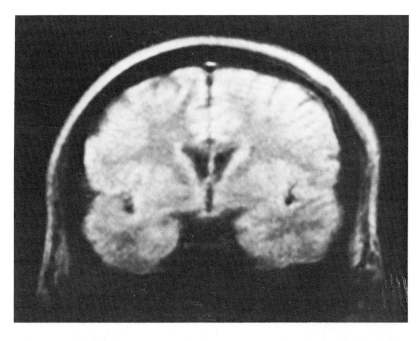

A

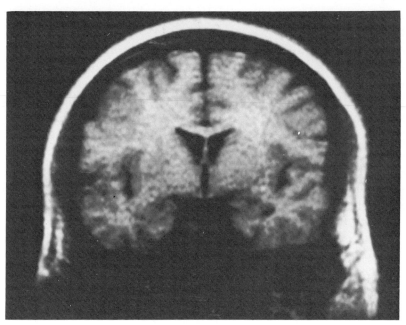

B

Figure 2-7. Partial saturation images. A, T_1 weighting with TR = 500 msec.
B, spin density weighting with TR = 2000 msec. The greater proton density
of gray matter relative to white matter increases gray matter intensity in the
long TR sequence and reduces white matter contrast.

the atoms are relatively fixed in space and the interactions giving rise to
T_2 tend to reinforce the decay process over time. In a liquid, molecular

motion occurs so rapidly that motion-induced fluctuations in the magnetic field average to nearly zero. Therefore, the values of T_2 are prolonged in the liquid. Many disease processes increase the water content of solid tissues, and thereby increase their T_2 values.

Scanning Methods

The MR signal contains more information about the tissues in which it originates than does the signal from any other imaging modality. Included in the signal is information about proton densities, spin-lattice relaxation times T_1, spin-spin relaxation times T_2, fluid flow, and spectral shifts associated with the bonding of hydrogen (or other elements) to specific molecules. By employing different scanning methods, certain aspects of this information can be isolated and depicted in an image or displayed as quantitative data. This flexibility is the major reason why MR presents such high potential — and challenge — to the investigator.

Pure spin density (i.e., proton density) images have limited usefulness. Furthermore, the relaxation times T_1 and T_2 are difficult to measure exactly. Consequently, methods that employ various combinations of proton density, T_1 and T_2 are employed most frequently in clinical imaging.

At least eight different imaging methods have been reported. However, the three most widely used are variants of the family of pulse techniques. All pulse imaging methods begin with the magnetization vector aligned with the magnetic field along the z axis. Then an rf pulse is applied to orient the vector away from the z axis and to induce precession. At a slightly later time, the first rf pulse is followed by one or more additional pulses, usually applied before relaxation is complete. Each imaging method utilizes a different combination of the first and succeeding pulses and in the time interval between them. These combinations yield images that emphasize one particular component of the tissue characteristics accessible to MR (spin density, T_1 or T_2).

Partial Saturation

The imaging method termed "partial saturation" (PS) consists of a series of equally spaced pulses, each of which rotates the magnetization vector through 90° (**Figure 2-8**). This technique also is referred to as "free induction decay" (FID) and as "saturation recovery" (SR). The latter expression should be reserved for the special case in which the magnetization vector recovers completely between successive rf pulses, however, and the former expression should be used to describe a single decay process when no repetitive rf pulses are used (1). Immediately following the first pulse in partial saturation, the magnetization vector lies in the xy plane and furnishes a maximum magnetic resonance (MR) signal. Spin-lattice and spin-spin relaxation then begin and

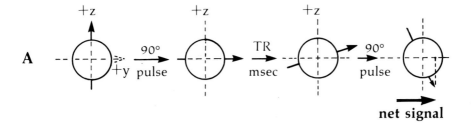

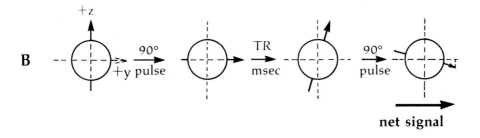

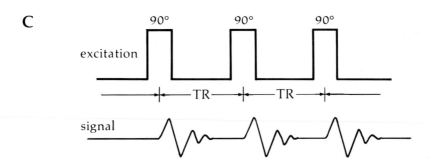

Figure 2-8. Partial saturation. A, regions with a long T_1 yield a small signal after the second 90° pulse because the magnetization vector relaxes just slightly in the +z direction between pulses. **B,** regions with a short T_1 relax nearly to +z between pulses; these regions yield a strong PS signal. The relative weights of spin density and T_1 relaxation in the image depend on the relationship of TR to TI. **C,** diagram of the partial saturation sequence.

the magnetization vector starts to relax toward the applied field (z axis) at different rates in different regions of the sample, according to the T_1 value of each region. Then, additional 90° pulses are applied and the signal is measured immediately after each. The interval between successive pulses is referred to as the "pulse repetition time TR." The second pulse causes the magnetization vector to rotate through another 90° arc; this time, however, the vector goes beyond the xy plane by an amount determined by the degree of relaxation occurring since the first pulse. In regions of tissue with short T_1, the vector returns to a position near the z axis between pulses, and then is carried slightly below the xy plane by the second pulse. In regions of long T_1, the vector returns only a short distance toward the z axis before the second pulse is applied and the second pulse carries the vector well beyond the xy plane. Since the strength of the MR signal from a region depends upon the component of the magnetization vector in the xy plane, the signal following the second pulse varies from one region to the next in a way that reflects the local T_1 value. (Because of the configuration of the receiver coil, only projections of the magnetization vector into the xy plane give rise to an MR signal.) The same process occurs following subsequent 90° pulses, leading eventually to an equilibrium condition with an rf signal of constant magnitude following each 90° pulse.

By increasing TR to a value greater than the average T_1 of the sample, PS images can be weighted by proton density to reveal the hydrogen content of the sample. With a long TR, the magnetizaton vector returns completely to the z axis between pulses, and is rotated exactly into the xy plane with each rf pulse to yield a maximum signal uncontaminated by relaxation effects. As described earlier, this technique is referred to as saturation recovery. With a shorter TR, the image is weighted by both proton density and relaxation times (principally T_1), leading usually to an enhancement of image contrast.

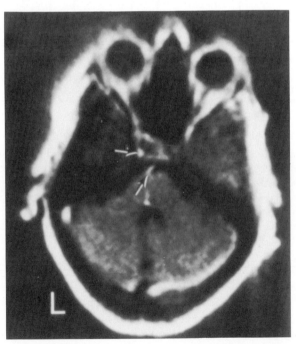

Figure 2-9. Obstruction of the right internal carotid artery: PS. The left internal carotid and basilar arteries are demonstrated in a moderate TR image (arrows), but the right internal carotid artery is not seen. A high signal intensity is produced by blood flow in the right transverse sinus and at the junction of the left sigmoid and transverse sinuses. (Reprinted with permission from Bydder, G.M., and others: Nuclear magnetic resonance imaging of the posterior fossa; 50 cases. Clin. Radiol. 34:173-188, 1983.)

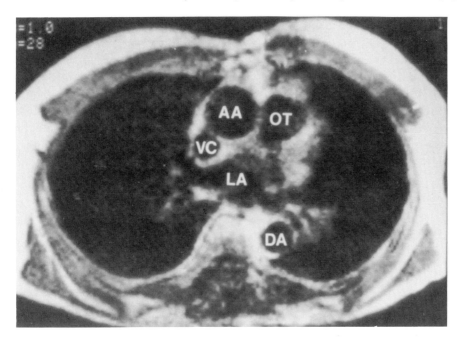

Figure 2-10. Non-gated transverse spin echo magnetic resonance image at the level of the base of the heart. The ascending aorta (AA), superior vena cava (VC), right ventricular outflow tract (OT), and left atrium (LA) are identified. These vascular structures are clearly visualized because flowing blood within their lumens produces little or no MR signal on images generated from the first spin echo (echo time [TE] = 28 msec). (Used with permission from Higgins, C.B., and others: Nuclear magnetic resonance imaging of the cardiovascular system. Radiographics 4:122-136, 1984.)

Partial saturation and other imaging methods can be made to reflect blood flow because blood flowing perpendicularly to the image section will partially or completely leave the section between rf pulses. This blood is replaced by blood with a magnetization vector aligned along the applied field because it has not been exposed to an rf pulse. An increased MR signal will emanate from this blood (**Figure 2-9**).

Rapid flow yields no signal from blood within vessels in two-pulse sequences such as inversion recovery and spin echo (**Figure 2-10**). Slow flow often yields increased signal from blood within vessels with these pulse sequences. The topic of MR signals from flowing fluids can be somewhat more complex than this simple explanation. The interested reader is referred to the literature for a more complete explanation.

Partial saturation scans with a short TR are also useful in highlighting regions with long T_1s, including cysts and subdural fluid collections.

Inversion Recovery

Inversion recovery (IR) imaging is a two-pulse sequence with many clinical applications. The first pulse is a 180° "inverting pulse" that rotates the magnetization vector from the +z axis onto the –z axis. Relaxation then occurs for a time TI, termed the interpulse delay time, before a second pulse is applied. During this interval the magnetization vector relaxes toward the +z axis at a rate determined by the local T_1 value. The second pulse is a 90° "read" pulse; the signal is measured immediately following this second pulse. After the repetition time TR, the entire process is repeated. Inversion recovery is diagrammed in **Figure 2-11**.

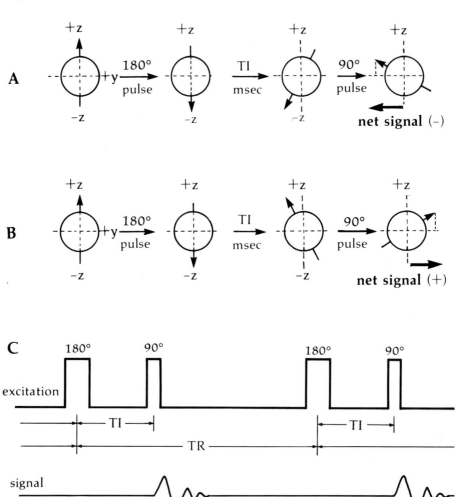

Figure 2-11. Inversion recovery. A, regions with a long T_1 yield a magnetization vector that relaxes only slightly toward the +z axis during the interpulse delay time TI. These regions yield a negative signal. **B,** regions with a short T_1 relax more and yield a positive signal. **C,** diagram of the inversion recovery sequence.

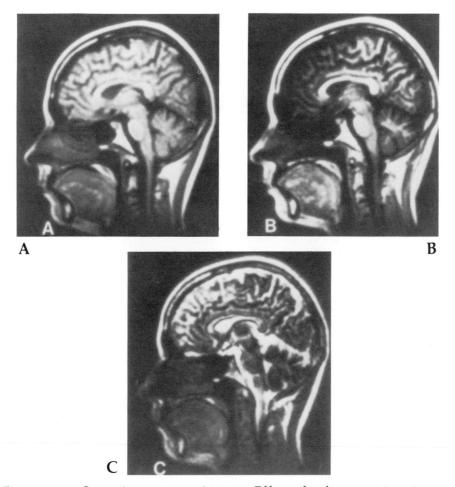

A   **B**

C

Figure 2-12. Inversion-recovery images. Effect of pulse repetition time on contrast. The images were obtained with an interpulse delay (TI) of 0.4 seconds. **A**, TR = 0.5 s. **B**, TR = 1 s. **C**, TR = 4 s. Contrast between white and gray matter increases with prolongation of the pulse repetition time. (Reprinted with permission from Wehrli, F.W., MacFall, J.R. and Newton, T.H.: Parameters determining the appearance of NMR images. Advanced Imaging Techniques, volume 2 in the Modern Neuroradiology series. Newton, T.H., and Potts, D.G., editors. San Anselmo: 1983, Clavadel Press.)

A magnetizaton vector that has relaxed quickly toward the +z axis because of a short T_1 is carried beyond the +z axis by the read pulse. Its projection into the xy plane is positive and so is the signal it generates, leading to a white appearance. A region of tissue with a long T_1 has a magnetization vector that relaxes only slightly before the read pulse. This vector falls short of the +z axis when the read pulse is applied, and its projection into the xy plane is negative, yielding a negative signal and a dark image. Inversion recovery images obtained at 0.3T for different values of the pulse repetition time TR are shown in **Figure 2-12.**

The relative signal amplitudes for white matter, gray matter, and cerebrospinal fluid (CSF) are plotted in **Figure 2-13** as a function of the interpulse delay time TI. Images for different values of the interpulse delay time TI are shown in **Figure 2-14**.

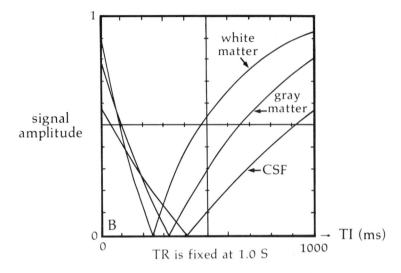

Figure 2-13. Signal intensity in the inversion recovery image. This graph exhibits three important features. **1**, negative MR signals are produced with short TI. However, most current imaging units detect the magnitude but not the sign of the MR signal. Hence, large negative signals are displayed with sign reversal as large positive signals to yield greater image brightness; less negative signals are displayed as smaller positive signals and reduced image brightness. Sign reversal leads to "reversed" image contrast; that is, regions of longer T_1 have increased image intensity compared to shorter T_1 regions. Gray matter is lighter than white matter with short TI intervals. **2**, as TI is increased from zero, the signal intensity progressively decreases, reaches zero, and then increases. The location where the signal is zero is called the "bounce point." This point occurs earlier in regions with shorter T_1 values. **3**, inversion recovery sequences commonly employ moderate or long TI intervals beyond the bounce point in most tissues. Contrast is "normal" with these parameters, and longer T_1 regions are displayed with decreased intensity.

Compared to PS images, IR images are weighted more heavily toward T_1 (2). They are useful particularly when high-image contrast is desired (e.g., in distinguishing white and gray matter in the brain). A variety of white matter diseases, tumors, and edema, have prolonged T_1s, and appear as dark regions in IR images. IR imaging may prove especially useful for the early detection of disease processes that involve white matter. Its discrimination of white matter tracts is also helpful in the localization of lesions that cause tract displacement.

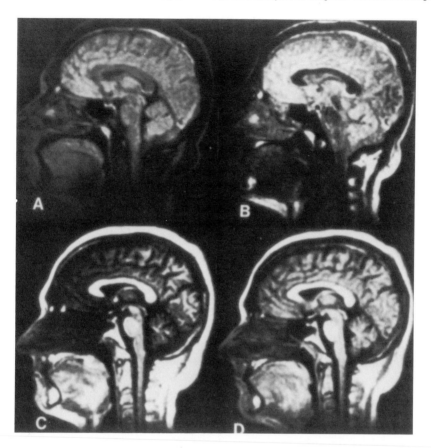

Figure 2-14. Inversion-recovery images. Effect of interpulse interval on contrast. These images were recorded from the same slice at a field strength of 0.3 tesla and a repetition time TR of 1 second. **A,** with a very short-TI interval image contrast is reversed and the shorter T_1 of the corpus callosum (white matter) yields a lower intensity signal compared to the adjacent gray matter. **B,** at a somewhat longer TI interval, the contrast between white and gray matter has increased, with the white matter yielding nearly zero signal intensity at this interpulse interval (the bounce point). CSF also has a slightly higher intensity than white matter because of its longer T_1. **C,** at a moderate TI interval, the contrast between white and gray matter is again prominent; the lower T_1 of white matter now yields a higher intensity signal compared to gray matter. **D,** at a somewhat longer TI interval, the contrast remains normal. (Reprinted with permission from Wehrli, F.W., MacFall, J.R. and Newton, T.H.: Parameters determining the appearance of NMR images. Advanced imaging Techniques, volume 2 in the Modern Neuroradiology series. Newton, T.H., and Potts, D.G., editors. San Anselmo: 1983, Clavadel Press.)

Spin Echo

Many disease processes produce a greater change in T_2 than in T_1. Spin-echo (SE) pulse sequences were developed specifically to demonstrate the spin-spin relaxation time T_2 (3). These sequences are often highly sensitive to the presence of pathology. In T_2 measurements, a problem arises because magnetic inhomogeneities of any kind produce spin dephasing. The inhomogeneities of interest arise from spin-spin interactions of nuclei; however, these inhomogeneities are weak compared to those from other sources. No magnet produces a completely homogeneous field, especially over a volume as large as the human

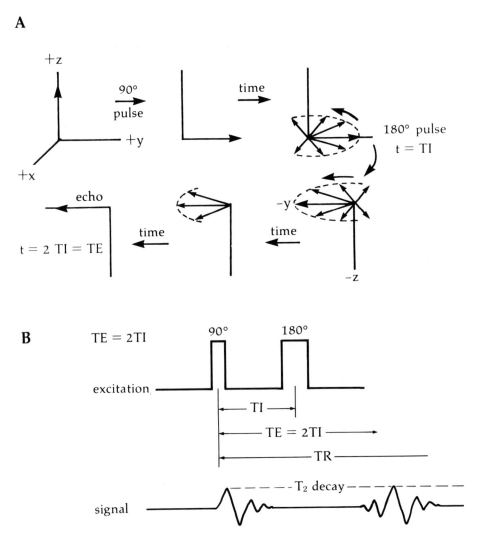

Figure 2-15. Formation of a spin echo. A, the magnetization vector begins to dephase after the initial (90°) rf pulse. Following the inverting pulse, the vector components at TE = 2TI converge to form an echo relatively free of machine-induced inhomogeneities. **B,** diagram of the spin-echo sequence.

body; even in the best magnets, variations in the magnetic field are much stronger than those caused by spin-spin interactions. In addition, the applied magnetic field is made even more inhomogeneous by application of additional magnetic fields needed for spatial information. In measurement of T_2, machine-induced inhomogeneities cause an artificial dephasing of the magnetization vector and must be neutralized so that only the magnetic inhomogeneities caused by spin-spin interactions in the tissue are observed.

The SE sequence begins with a 90° pulse to rotate the magnetization vector into the xy plane (**Figure 2-15**). Magnetic field inhomogeneities then cause the vector to dephase into components in various orientations in the xy plane. After an interpulse delay time TI, which is so short that little T_1 relaxation occurs, a second pulse is applied to rotate the components through 180°. After rotation, components of the magnetization vector that had been diverging in the direction of faster spin (counter-clockwise) are positioned to converge upon the other components. These components still represent regions where the magnetic field is more intense and hence are still precessing faster. Similarly, regions that are precessing more slowly are positioned ahead of the other components of the magnetization vector after inversion. These components continue to precess more slowly. After rotation, the continued counterclockwise motion of the faster components now closes the dephasing fan instead of widening it, and the components converge to reconstitute the original signal or, more properly, its 180° "echo" (**Figure 2-15**). This reconstruction occurs over a time 2TI = TE, since the components of the vector take just as long to converge as they did to diverge. (TE is the time between maximum signals in a repeated spin-echo pulse sequence.) In the spin-echo technique, the machine-generated magnetic inhomogeneities act as long in one direction as in the other, and they cancel. Spin-spin interactions among nuclei, however, produce fluctuating inhomogeneities that cannot be cancelled with any degree of precision.

In the spin-echo technique, successive echoes are generated by applying additional 180° pulses, a process known as the Carr-Purcell (CP) sequence (**Figure 2-16**). The magnetization vectors that come together to form each new echo are given more time for spin-spin interaction; this time causes them to fan out in a way that is not neutralized by the spin echo process. A "snapshot" of the magnetization vectors at the return of each echo shows a progressive dephasing due to true spin-spin relaxation, independent of machine-generated inhomogeneities. Since the reduction in signal intensity between echoes is due mainly to true spin-spin relaxation, measurement of the relative strengths of two successive echoes allows T_2 to be estimated. The accuracy of this estimate improves as the number of 180° pulses used in the computation increases.

excitation

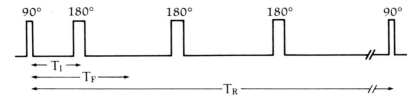

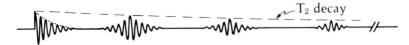

detection

Figure 2-16. Multiple echo sequence and timing diagram. The 180° pulses follow at times TI, 3TI, 5TI, 7 TI, and the echoes appear at times 2TI = TE, 2TE, 3TE, 4TE. The echo envelope (dashed line) decays with a time constant T_2, the true spin-spin relaxation time.

To reduce the cumulative effects of inhomogeneities in the Carr-Purcell sequence, a modification is employed in which selected phase shifts are introduced between the 90° pulse and the series of 180° pulses. Alternatively, the modifications can be introduced between the 180° rf pulses. The use of these modifications is referred to as a Carr-Purcell-Meiboom-Gill (CPMG) sequence.

The clinical application of spin-echo sequences presents the user with several options. The intensity of the SE signal is influenced by several factors, including the local spin density and T_1 and T_2 values, as well as the TE and TR intervals chosen for the examination. Tissue contrast is determined largely by the TE and TR intervals selected as a reflection of the T_1 and T_2 values of the tissues. The importance of choosing the proper TR and TE values is illustrated in **Figure 2-17**.

Applications of the spin-echo technique to clinical imaging can be simplified by considering three categories of TR and TE intervals: short, moderate, and long (Table 2). If a moderate TE interval is chosen for spin-echo imaging, regions with short T_2 values will dephase prior to echo reception and yield little signal intensity. These regions will appear dark in the image (**Figure 2-18**). Regions with longer values of T_2

Table 2

Classification of pulse intervals

	Short	Moderate	Long
TR	0.4-1.1 T_1	1.1-2.4 T_1	2.4-4 T_1
TE	10-30 msec	30-60 msec	60-100 msec
TI(IR)	0.2-0.7 T_1	0.7-1.5 T_1	1.5-2.5 T_1

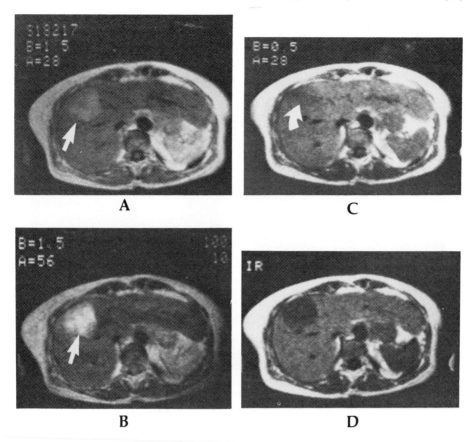

Figure 2-17. Liver metastasis: spin echo. A, the metastasis has a prolonged T_1 and is imaged with decreased intensity in inversion recovery. **B,** the metastasis also has a prolonged T_2 and is imaged with decreased intensity in a moderate TR/moderate TE spin echo image. **C,** in a moderate TR/short TE sequence there is less accentuation of long T_2 regions and the intensity of the lesion is decreased compared to **B. D,** the lesion is nearly isointense compared to normal liver in a short TR/short TE sequence because of the opposing effects on image intensity of the prolonged T_1 and T_2 values, and the increased T_1 weighting in this sequence compared to **B** and **C.** A lesion that is isointense with normal tissue at one TE interval often can be distinguished in an image with a different TE interval. Images with different TE intervals can be obtained during a single examination by using a string of 180° pulses, each of which generates an echo. Usually, the first echo corresponds to a short TE interval, the second echo to a moderate TE interval, and so on. This procedure does not increase imaging time significantly since TE usually is much shorter than TR. (Reprinted with permission from Moss, A.A., and others: Liver, gallbladder, alimentary tube, spleen, peritoneal cavity, and pancreas. In Margulis, A.R., and others, editors: Clinical Magnetic Resonance Imaging. San Francisco: 1983, Radiology Research and Education Foundation.)

will remain largely in phase and yield an intense echo. These regions will appear light in the image. Regions with T_2 values near the TE interval chosen will be displayed with intermediate intensities. If a short TE interval is chosen, regions with moderate and long T_2 values

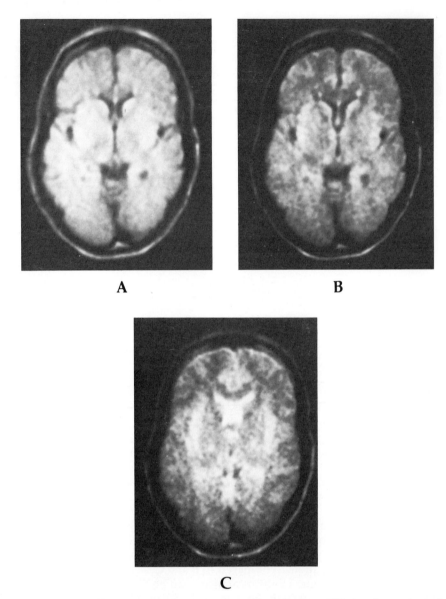

Figure 2-18. Effect on image contrast of changing TE in the spin-echo sequence. The same section of normal brain is shown with **A**, short TE, **B**, moderate TE, and **C**, long TE parameters. Moderate TR intervals were used for each image and there is moderate T_1 weighting. Cerebrospinal fluid (CSF) is dark in **A** and **B** because of its long T_1 and is bright in **C** because the long TE interval accentuates the long T_2 of CSF. There is little white-gray matter discrimination in **A** because the short T_1 and T_2 values of white matter have opposing effects on white matter intensity relative to gray matter, thereby neutralizing contrast. Increasing the TE interval increases white-gray matter contrast by accentuating T_2 differences, with white matter becoming less intense than gray matter because of its shorter T_2. The long TE image, **C**, has increased noise compared to **A**. (Reprinted with permission from Bydder, G.M., and others: Clinical NMR imaging of the brain: 140 cases, Am. J. Roentgenol. 139:215-236, 1982.)

will remain largely in phase, and both will appear bright in the SE image; regions with short T_2 will be displayed with lower intensity. A long TE interval yields images in which only regions of long T_2 remain bright, with short and moderate T_2 regions appearing dark. Long TE sequences highlight pathology by emphasizing regions with prolonged T_2 values. However, the overall intensity is reduced with longer TE intervals because complete spin-spin relaxation will have occurred in much of the tissue. Hence, long TE images are often noisy and provide rather poor lesion resolution.

One difficulty in categorizing TI intervals in inversion recovery, or TR intervals in any of the pulse sequences, is that the influence of the intervals on tissue contrast depends on the average T_1 of the tissue. Since T_1 varies with magnetic field strength, identical TR or TI intervals will yield different contrast characteristics in images from different MR units. Approximate values of T_1 are shown in Table 3 for gray and white matter for three magnetic field strengths covering the range of current imaging units. Unlike T_1, proton density and T_2 are tissue characteristics that do not vary significantly with magnetic field strength. For a variety of tissues T_2 falls between 60 and 120 msec, with a value of about 115 msec for gray matter and 80 msec for white matter. T_2 values for fluid collections are somewhat longer; for example, T_2 is approximately 150 msec for cerebrospinal fluid.

Table 3
Approximate values of T_1 over the range of
magnetic field strengths used in current MRI units

		0.15T	0.5T	1.5T
Gray Matter	T_1	500 msec	600 msec	800 msec
White Matter	T_1	350 msec	400 msec	600 msec

The purpose of the TR interval is to provide time for the magnetic moment to become realigned along the z axis at the end of each pulse sequence. If this realignment is incomplete in any region of tissue, the signal intensity from the region is diminished in the next sequence. Local T_1 values determine the rate at which different regions recover their magnetization, with the magnetization recovering sooner in regions of shorter T_1. Long TR intervals provide sufficient time for realignment to occur throughout the tissue and minimize the influence of T_1 differences on image contrast. Hence, long TR images exhibit reduced T_1 weighting, and contrast is determined by regional differences in spin density and T_2.

During short and moderate TR intervals, some magnetization vectors do not realign completely with the z axis, with fewer realigning during short TR than during moderate TR sequences. These images are weighted more toward T_1, with longer T_1 regions exhibiting decreased intensity. With a short TR interval, incomplete realignment of some magnetization vectors reduces the overall intensity of the MR signal. Therefore, although short TR spin-echo images accentuate T_1 contrast, they also yield somewhat noisier images that may increase the difficulty of visualizing subtle lesions.

Increasing TR makes it possible to image additional sections in multiplanar imaging. Theoretically, twice as many sections could be examined during the same scan if the TR interval were doubled; of course, the examination time would also be doubled. Long TR sequences may be used when many sections are needed to image a portion of the body. For example, long TR images are well-suited to transverse imaging of the brain; on the other hand, short TR images yield a sufficient number of sections for sagittal brain imaging. The use of separate short and long TR sequences can yield images with different degrees of T_1 and T_2 weighting in different planes.

Making an Image

The encoding of an MR signal with spatial information is one of the more complex aspects of magnetic resonance imaging. The task of understanding the encoding process is complicated further by the practice by different manufacturers of using different methods. The methods described here illustrate the principles involved; most manufacturers use some combination of these principles.

In the MR unit, the imaging plane may be selected by applying an alternating magnetic field perpendicular to the main magnetic field. The alternating field causes the total magnetic field at most points to vary with time (**Figure 2-19**). In response, the frequency of the MR signal from these points varies with time, increasing as the field

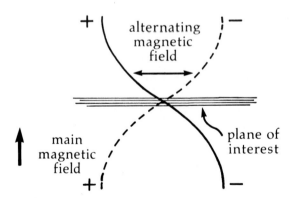

Figure 2-19. How a section of tissue may be selected for imaging. An alternating magnetic field causes the resonance frequency at most points to change with time. The magnetic field and resonance frequency are unaltered only at "nodal points," which lie in the section of interest. The signal from this plane can be electronically extracted from the rest of the signals by filtering out components that vary with time.

increases and decreasing as the field decreases. At "nodal" points in a narrow zone that defines the region of interest, the total magnetic field remains constant and the signal frequency does not vary with time. By filtering out signal components that vary with time, the signal from the region of interest can be extracted. By electronically moving the nodal point while changing the direction of the applied gradient, contiguous transaxial, sagittal, or coronal (or other) images can be obtained without ever moving the patient.

The method described above is seldom used any longer in clinical MR. A more popular method of plane selection is to apply a smaller additional magnetic field (called a gradient) across the sample. The gradient is designed so that it reinforces the main field on one side, subtracts from it on the other side, varies smoothly in between, and does not change with time. The gradient alters the field only along one axis, and the magnetic field remains constant in each plane perpendicular to the direction of the gradient. The magnetic field, and therefore the resonance frequency, is different in adjacent planes perpendicular to the gradient. Hence, an rf pulse with a narrow, "selective" range of frequencies affects only the tissue in a single planar section. That is, only the protons in this section are excited; no signal emanates from other sections of the tissue. This process is called "selective irradiation" (**Figure 2-20**).

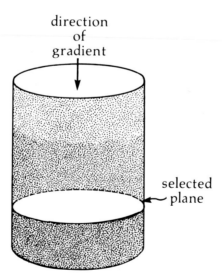

direction
of
gradient

selected
plane

Figure 2-20. Plane selection by selective irradiation. A magnetic gradient is added to the main magnetic field, causing it to vary smoothly from one end of the sample to the other. In any plane perpendicular to the gradient, all points experience the same magnetic field and have the same resonance frequency. Adjacent planes experience different magnetic fields and have different resonance frequencies. rf pulses with a narrow range of frequencies induce resonance only in the plane with the appropriate resonance frequency.

Once a section is selected, further manipulations of magnetic gradients separate the signals from different points in the section. A second gradient can be applied across the section of interest so that it adds to the field on one side and subtracts from it on the other. The main magnetic field is unaltered only along a line perpendicular to the direction of the gradient (**Figure 2-21**, central line). Lines parallel to the central line in the image section will yield an MR signal of higher or lower frequency compared to that of the central line. When signals are received, they are separated into different frequencies, where each frequency represents the signal from a particular line in the section. At each frequency, the signal intensity represents the contribution of all points in a line parallel to the central line. The representation of a signal from a line as a single value in a distribution of frequencies is a type of projection. By electronically rotating the magnetic field gradient around the patient in the section of interest, these data can be reconstructed into an image. The reconstruction technique is analogous to the image reconstruction process used in CT. In MR it is called zeugmatography, the first reconstruction process used in MR. (This expression conveys the coupling of the static and gradient magnetic fields used in MR with the rf pulse used to elicit the MR signal.)

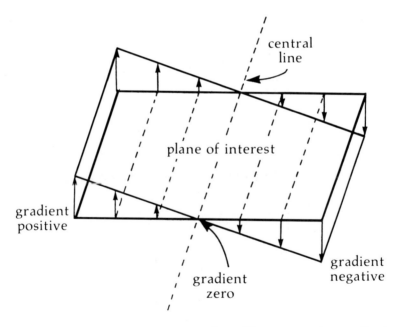

Figure 2-21. Projection reconstruction. The magnetic gradient applied across the plane of interest is positive (adds to the main magnetic field) on one side and negative (subtracts from the main field) on the other. The main magnetic field is unaltered along the central line. Each line has a frequency characteristic of a particular magnetic field intensity, and each point on the line contributes to the strength of the signal at that frequency. Rotating the gradient leads to a series of projections that can be reconstructed into an image.

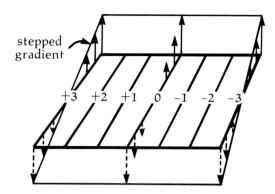

stepped
gradient

+3 +2 +1 0 −1 −2 −3

Figure 2-22. Two-dimensional Fourier transformation. A plane is selected and a gradient applied, as shown in Figure 2-20. Line "zero" is the central line. The other lines are numbered to indicate the strength of the gradient. A second gradient (shown) is applied perpendicular to the first and introduces a phase shift in the signal from each line. The second gradient is increased stepwise for subsequent pulse sequences while the first gradient remains fixed. Fourier transformation of the MR data then yields an image.

A much more common reconstruction method in MR is the two-dimensional Fourier Transformation (2DFT) (4). A fixed gradient is applied to the selected image plane, and a second perpendicular gradient is applied briefly (**Figure 2-22**). The effect of the second gradient is to momentarily speed up or slow down the precession in each line defined by the fixed gradient. Along a given line, each magnetization vector rotates faster or slower, depending on its position. This process introduces phase differences among vectors at different points in the line; hence, each point is localized in terms of an x coordinate described by phase and a y coordinate identified by the resonance frequency. Increasing the strength of the second gradient in many small steps during a scan eventually provides the computer with enough information to perform a Fourier transformation and make an image. This particular imaging technique is free of the linear type of motion artifact common in CT images. Instead, the 2DFT technique introduces a generalized blurring, and occasional minor ring artifacts, in the image when motion is present, sometimes accompanied by minor vertical streaks.

The same principles can be extended to a three-dimensional Fourier transformation process, which permits simultaneous collection of data from an entire volume of sample. Each volume element (voxel) in the data set is a 1 to 2 mm cube, whereas the voxel size of planar methods is 1 to 2 mm square in the plane of interest and of selectable thickness in the depth dimension. The principal advantage of the volume imaging method is that once the data have been collected, they can be dissected into 1 to 2 mm thick slices in any orientation, provided that computer storage is adequate. In planar methods, a separate scan is required for each orientation. Both planar and volume reconstruction methods are employed in commercial MR units. Because of the significantly longer data collection time for the volume imaging method, the 2DFT planar method is more common.

Imaging Times

Imaging times are significantly longer in MR than in CT, primarily because the MR signal is weak and easily obscured by noise. (Noise is any information present in the data acquisition process that does not contribute to the desired image.) To extract the MR signal from noise, it is necessary to repeat the rf pulse sequences several times for each projection. The principal sources of noise are commercial radio stations, fluorescent lights, electric motors, electrical connections and microprocessors within the MR equipment, and thermal noise from within the patient. The external sources of noise can be reduced by enclosing the imaging unit in a copper-clad room and by installing electronic filters to remove low-frequency (e.g., 60 Hz) noise. Electrical connections can be replaced by optical coupling devices. It is much more difficult to control noise from the patient, and this source is now the limiting factor in noise considerations for MR imaging. Evidence suggests that increasing the intensity of the magnetic field increases the strength, as well as the frequency, of the MR signal; hence, higher magnetic field intensities may permit the use of shorter imaging times because fewer repetitions of the rf pulse sequences are required to obtain an adequate signal. Current scanners operate with static magnetic field strengths from 0.07 to 1.5 tesla (0.7 to 15 kilogauss). Improvements in the design of rf transmitting and receiving antennas may help reduce scan times somewhat, but significant progress in shortening scan times probably will come slowly. A more significant improvement has evolved from techniques to collect data sequentially for many slices. That is, data are collected for each slice during the pulse repetition times of the other slices in the volume of interest (**Figure 2-23**). These multi-slice techniques are now available with most commercial MR units.

The relationship between the strength of a signal and the magnitude of the noise is often described as the signal-to-noise (S/N) ratio. As described above, this ratio is much lower for MR than for alternate modalities of imaging. Consequently, tissues must be sampled repetitively to obtain enough data to separate the signal from noise, and imaging times are long for MR compared to other modalities. Since the signal increases approximately linearly with magnetic field intensity, whereas the noise increases more slowly, improved S/N ratios are obtained in higher magnetic fields, and imaging times can be reduced somewhat. High S/N ratios also permit the imaging of thinner sections of tissue, and also facilitate high-resolution magnified ("zoom") images of small regions. The advantages of a higher S/N ratio are among the

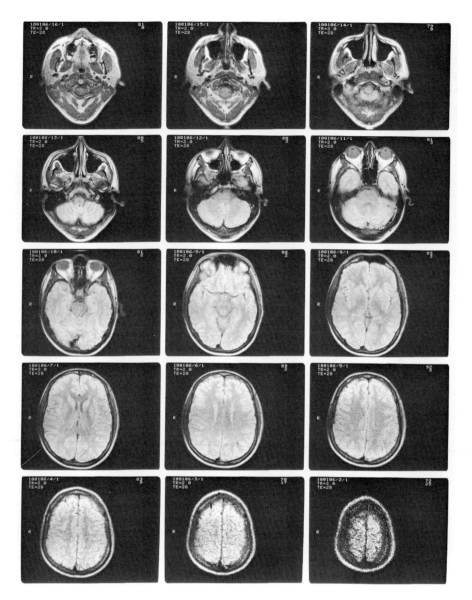

Figure 2-23. Multi-slice SE images. Fifteen images were obtained in 6.5 minutes (0.35T; TE = 28 msec; TR = 2 sec).

major reasons for purchasing an imaging unit operating at 1T and above. Among the disadvantages of a high-field strength system are difficulties in obtaining multiple images of different sections simultaneously because of limitations in rf coil design, and some loss of image contrast caused by a reduction in differences in T_1 among tissues at higher field strengths.

Many disease processes produce changes in more than one MR parameter (e.g., many processes affect both T_1 and T_2). That is, MR has

41

several "windows" through which abnormalities can be detected. To detect a lesion and characterize it in terms of changes in T_1 and T_2, sets of images are required with different settings for the imaging parameters (TR, TI, TE, etc.). From these data, values for T_1 and T_2 can be extracted mathematically. The accuracy of these values improves as more data sets are compiled for their extraction. The accuracy also depends on the actual values of T_1 and T_2; longer relaxation times are more difficult to estimate because the data used in the computation are noisier (5). A complete MR examination, with computation of T_1 and T_2 values, could take as much as 20 to 40 minutes for completion. One major avenue of current research in MR is the appearance of various disease processes in different images, so that eventually protocols can be established to tailor scan techniques to particular clinical indications (6).

References

1. American College of Radiology, *Glossary of NMR Terms*. Chicago: 1983, The College.

2. Wehrli, F.W., MacFall, J.R., and Newton, T.H.: *Parameters determining the appearance of NMR images. Advanced imaging Techniques*, Volume 2 in the Modern Neuroradiology series. Newton, T.H., and Potts, D.G., editors. San Anselmo: 1983, Clavadel Press.

3. Harms, S.E., and others: Principles of nuclear magnetic resonance imaging. Radiographics 4:26-43, 1984.

4. Kumar, A., Welti, I., and Ernst, R.R.: NMR Fourier zeugmatography. J. Mag. Reson. 18:69-83, 1975.

5. Buonanno, F.S., and others: Proton NMR imaging in experimental ischemic infarction. Stroke 14:178-184, 1983.

6. Hendee, W.R., and Morgan, C.R.: Magnetic resonance imaging. Western J. Med. In press.

Chapter 3
Biological Effects

One of the major advantages often quoted for MR is the production of clinical images without the use of ionizing radiation. Although this advantage has considerable appeal to referring physicians, patients, and the public in general, it is of questionable significance when evaluated objectively. When performed properly, imaging techniques employing ionizing radiation also pose little risk to patients undergoing diagnostic examination. For this reason, the success of MR ultimately will depend on its contributions to the detection and diagnosis of disease, rather than on its hazard relative to other imaging modalities (1).

During an MR examination the patient is not exposed to ionizing radiation. Still, MR must be evaluated in terms of any potential risks to the patient associated with its use. The risks of MR are labeled "potential risks" because no bioeffects have been identified for the magnetic fields employed in magnetic resonance imaging. The potential risks are associated with the three types of magnetic fields employed in MR: (1) the static magnetic field used to align the magnetic moments, (2) the time-varying magnetic fields used to extract positional information within the tissues, and (3) the magnetic field associated with the pulse of radiofrequency energy transmitted into the body to elicit MR signals. Possible bioeffects associated with each of these fields are considered in this chapter.

Static Magnetic Fields

Many experiments have been performed to study the biological effects of exposure of cells and animals to static magnetic fields of relatively high intensity. These experiments have often yielded nondefinitive or controversial results. In some cases, the experiments have not been repeatable by other investigators. One effect is abnormal electrocardiographic tracings measured in animals placed in intense magnetic fields. In all likelihood, these findings are caused by small voltages induced across blood vessels as blood flows through the vessels at right angles to the applied magnetic field. These small voltages are thought to be inconsequential to patient welfare. One would be concerned about this "magnetic hydrodynamic effect" on the heart and great vessels only if the magnetic field strengths or the velocities of blood flow were much greater than those encountered during MR. In animal studies of this effect, Gaffey and Tenforde (2) noted that: no arrythmias or alterations in heart rate are induced; the normal EKG resumes immediately when exposure to high magnetic fields is terminated; and no changes in blood chemistry or blood pressure are observed in the animals. At the field strengths employed in current NMR imaging units, no changes in EKG tracings have been noted in volunteers undergoing imaging procedures (3).

Budinger (4) has proposed the following four possible mechanisms whereby magnetic fields might influence biological processes or organism behavior.

1. Reorientation of macromolecules leading to changes in chemical kinetics and membrane permeability. Certain molecules such as DNA and cellular subunits such as retinal rods and sickled red cells have magnetic properties that vary with direction. These entities are said to exhibit magnetic susceptibility anisotropy; in a magnetic field they experience a twisting force or torque. This effect is not considered biologically important at magnetic field strengths below about 2T.

2. Changes in enzyme kinetics caused by the quenching of superconductivity present in some organic molecules. For these molecules, superconductivity has been proposed as an important factor in reaction kinetics. Magnetic fields can cause a substance to lose its superconducting property. This loss could affect the rate of enzyme reactions. The effect, however, is not expected to occur at field strengths below 20T or so.

3. Reductions in the velocity of nerve conduction. The conduction of nerve impulses is similar to the conduction of electric current in a wire; in a magnetic field the current velocity in the nerve may be affected. However, magnetic field intensities of 20T or more probably are required to produce changes in nerve conduction velocity.

4. Superposition of low voltages on natural biopotentials. This effect is discussed above in terms of EKG changes induced by small potential differences induced across blood vessels in a magnetic field. The effect is not expected, and has not been seen, at magnetic field strengths below 2T.

To determine if magnetic fields induce genetic changes or impair the development of the fetus, Mahlum and co-workers (5) conducted a series of experiments on mice with static magnetic fields of 1T. No effects of either type were demonstrable.

Time-Varying Magnetic Fields

In MR instruments, time-varying magnetic fields are used to localize the origin of the MR signal. These variations in magnetic field intensity can induce electric currents in body tissues. If the currents are intense enough, they can stimulate certain body tissues such as nerve cells and muscle fibers in the heart and the respiratory musculature. However, the rate of change in magnetic field intensity required to produce observable effects such as heart fibrillation are far above those employed in MR. During long exposure times, activation of platelets has been observed; a more definitive study of this process is needed.

At much lower rates of change in magnetic field intensity, visual light flashes can be induced. These visual changes, described as magnetic phosphenes, were described almost a century ago by d'Arsonval (6). Although under certain conditions phosphenes can be induced at relatively low rates of change in magnetic intensity, no permanent deleterious effects are thought to be associated with this phenomenon.

Radiofrequency Magnetic Field

The radiofrequency energy pulses used to elicit MR signals from a region of tissue do not cause cellular stimulation in the manner of the lower frequency time-varying magnetic fields discussed above. Instead, the effect of exposure of tissue to a radiofrequency field is simple tissue heating caused by absorption of energy from the incident field. This principle is employed in the therapeutic application of short-wave diathermy.

The basal metabolic rate of humans averages about 1-5 W/kg during sleep and as much as 15 W/kg during heavy exercise. Absorption of energy at a rate of 1 W/kg continuously for an hour would raise temperatures by about 1°C in tissues with little or no blood supply, such as the testes and the lens of the eye (7). Other tissues would experience a smaller increase in temperature. Recently, the American National Standards Institute (ANSI) proposed an average whole body limit at 0.4 W/kg, with a maximum energy absorption in any tissue of 8 W/kg. Power dissipation from MR units is expected to be well below these limits. For example, Edelstein and associates (8) have demonstrated that the maximum time-averaged absorbed power from typical MR units is below 1 W/kg and often less than 0.1 W/kg when averaged over the exposed region of tissue.

A few nonthermal effects of the radiofrequency magnetic field have been studied. These studies have been conducted at levels exceeding those employed in MR, and have yielded controversial results. Radiofrequency energy in the frequency range of 1 to 75 Hz apparently can affect the binding of calcium ions, resulting possibly in a change in the stimulus threshold of nerve tissue (9). At relatively high-power densities, certain particles such as charcoal, starch, milk, and blood cells will align to form chains parallel to the electric lines of force. This effect is termed the "bead-chain effect," and probably is caused by the induction of charges on the particles by the radiofrequency field. The effect occurs only at field intensities above those causing a heating effect. At very high frequencies and relatively high specific energy absorption, some investigators have reported changes in the permeability of the blood-brain barrier in animals (10-12), presumably as a secondary effect of alterations in blood flow, blood pressure, or blood vessel area.

Prosthetic Implants

Metal objects embedded in tissue will absorb more energy than the surrounding tissue because of the increased conductivity of the metal. For small objects such as surgical clips, the heating effect should be negligible; for larger metallic objects such as those used in hip prostheses, the temperature of surrounding tissues could be increased by a few degrees. (13).

Artificial Cardiac Pacemakers

In the presence of relatively weak magnetic fields, some types of cardiac pacemakers may function in unpredictable ways (14). For this reason, patients with cardiac pacemakers have not been imaged to date in MR units, at least in the United States or in Great Britain. In addition, care is taken to exclude patients with cardiac pacemakers from the immediate environment surrounding an MR unit.

Pregnancy

There is no experimental evidence to suggest that the embryo or fetus is particularly sensitive to the magnetic fields employed in MR. Nevertheless, concern has been expressed over possible fetal effects, and consequently few installations have examined pregnant patients. Because of the absence of ionizing radiation, MR may be inherently more acceptable than x-ray and nuclear medicine techniques for examining the fetus. It is conceivable that MR may someday be competitive with ultrasound for certain types of fetal examinations.

Human Epidemiological Studies

Few studies are available of the possible effects of magnetic fields on human physiology and behavior. Studies that are available are more anecdotal than comprehensive, principally because the number of individuals available for study is small and because the studies to date are retrospective rather than prospective.

Beischer studied physicists and technicians working in magnetic fields up to 2T for a few days per year and concluded that no health effects were apparent (15). A few years ago Russian scientists reported that 1,600 workers whose hands were exposed to field strengths of 35 to 50 mT experienced symptoms of headache, fatigue, hand swelling, and skin desquamation. These experiences have not been reproducible in facilities in the western world.

Summary

Several hypothetical biological effects are associated with the exposure of humans to the types of magnetic fields employed in MR. However, computations and limited experimental data suggest that these effects are not detectable at the field strengths used for imaging. Hence, the principal concerns of MR are possible tissue heating effects associated with large metallic protheses, influences on the operation of cardiac pacemakers, and the remote possibility that a fetus may somehow be peculiarly sensitive to magnetic fields. More practical concerns include the hazardous nature of flying metal objects carried into the environment of an MR unit, the experience of claustrophobia in 5% or so of patients examined in clinical MR units, and the occasional difficulty in caring for acutely ill patients during an MR examination. With proper design of an imaging facility and careful selection of patients for examination, however, it appears that MR can be conducted with a high degree of patient safety.

References

1. Hendee, W.R.: The advantage of no radiation exposure. Appl. Radiol. 11:6:146, 1982.
2. Gaffey, C.T., and Tenforde, T.S.: Alterations in the rat electrocardiogram induced by stationary magnetic fields. Berkeley: 1981, University of California, Lawrence Berkeley Laboratory.
3. Saunders, R.D.: Biologic effects of NMR clinical imaging. Appl. Radiol. Sept./Oct. 43-46, 1982.
4. Budinger, T.F.: Nuclear magnetic resonance (NMR) in vivo studies: known thresholds for health effects. J. Comput. Assist. Tomog. 5:800-811, 1981.
5. Mahlum, D.D., Sikov, M.R., and Dicker, J.R.: Dominant lethal studies in mice exposed to direct current magnetic fields. In *Biological Effects of Extremely Low Frequency Electro-Magnetic Fields.* Proc. 18th Hanford Life Sciences Symp., Richland, WA 1978, NTIS-CONF 781016, 1979, 474-484.
6. d'Arsonval, M.A.: Dispositifs pour la mesure des courants alternatifs a toutes frequences. Comput. Rad. Seances. Soc. Biol. Ses. Fil. 3:451, 1896.
7. American National Standards Institute (ANSI) Draft C95.1, Standard microwave news. 1:5-6, 1981.

8. Edelstein, W.A., and others: NMR imaging at 5.1 MHz: Work in progress. Proc. Int. Symp. Nuc. Mag. Reson. Imag. 139-145, 1981.

9. Tenforde, T.S.: Thermal aspects of electromagnetic field interaction with bound calcium ions at the nerve cell surface. J. Theor. Biol. 83:517-521, 1980.

10. Oscar, K.J., and Hawkins, T.D.: Microwave alteration of the blood-brain barrier system of rats. Brain Res. 126:281-292, 1977.

11. Albert, E.N.: Light and electron microscopic observations on the blood-brain barrier after microwave radiation. In: Proc. of Symp. on Biological Effects and Measurements of Radiofrequency/ Microwaves. DHEW, Rockville, MD, 1977, 294-304.

12. Oscar, K.J., and others: Local cerebral blood flow after microwave exposure. Brain Res. 204:220-225, 1981.

13. Davis, P.L., and others: Potential hazards in NMR imaging: Heating effects of changing magnetic fields and RF fields on small metallic implants. Am. J. Roentgenol. 137:857-860, 1981.

14. Bridges, J.E., and Frazier, M.J.: The effects of 60 Hz electric and magnetic field on implanted cardiac pacemakers. EPRI EA-1174. Proj. 079-1, 1979.

15. Beischer, D.E.: Human tolerance to magnetic fields. Astronautics 7:24, 1982.

Chapter 4
Design of a Magnetic Resonance Unit

In the evolution of the clinical applications of magnetic resonance, many imaging techniques have been proposed, and different manufacturers have pursued alternate pathways in the design of their imaging units. In all likelihood, none of the pathways currently available will be an optimum solution for all MR applications, and modifications to the design of at least some commercial units can be expected as more are installed in clinical environments around the world.

In spite of the variability among MR units, some common elements can be identified. For example, an MR imaging unit can be separated into six major subsystems (**Figure 4-1**). The subsystems are:

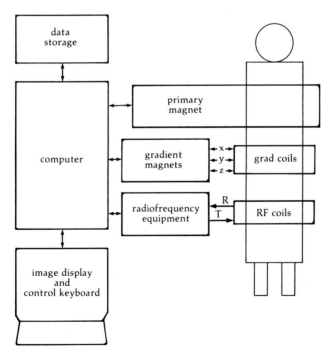

Figure 4-1. A simplified schematic of an MR unit showing the six basic subsystems: primary magnet, gradient magnet and coils, radiofrequency equipment, computer, data storage and data display. (Modified with permission received from: Fullerton, G.D.: Basic concepts of NMR imaging. Mag. Res. May 1, 1982, 39-53.)

(1) primary magnet

(2) magnetic gradient

(3) radiofrequency equipment

(4) computer

(5) data storage

(6) display unit

Each of these subsystems is described below.

Primary Magnet

The primary magnet supplies the static magnetic field for MR imaging, and its characteristics are critical to obtaining satisfactory images. One of the most important characteristics is the uniformity of the magnetic field, because slight nonuniformities produce image distortion and artifacts. For units intended solely for proton imaging, the magnetic field should be uniform to 1 part in 10^5 in the region where the patient is positioned for examination. For **in vivo** spectroscopic applications, the specifications for field uniformity will be more strict by at least an order of magnitude.

Three types of primary magnets are used in MR units: resistive magnets, operating up to about 0.15T; permanent magnets, operating at field strengths up to 0.3T; and superconductive systems, above 0.15T. Each of these magnet types generates a magnetic field that is many thousands of times stronger than the earth's magnetic field.

Resistive magnets utilize significant amounts of electrical power to maintain the magnetic field, and must be water-cooled to remove the heat generated by the dissipated electricity. Resistive magnets cost about $100,000, operate with relatively few problems, and produce magnetic fields that are somewhat less stable and homogeneous than those from superconducting systems (Table 4). These systems yield high-quality images, but are expensive to operate because of their power consumption.

Superconducting magnets consist of a cylindrical coil of niobium-tin alloy wires embedded in a copper matrix and surrounded by a vacuum dewar. They cost more than $200,000, produce exceptionally stable and homogeneous fields, and yield somewhat better spatial resolution and soft tissue contrast. They also are less expensive to operate, even though they must be cooled to within a few degrees of absolute zero by liquid helium. They draw no electrical current once the magnetic field is established. Although manufacturers have considerable experience building large superconducting magnets, the units still are not entirely immune from potential problems. For example, a vacuum leak could cause a slight rise in temperature of the windings and lead to a sudden loss of superconductivity (quenching). Heat generated by the circulating current as it suddenly encounters electrical

Table 4

Magnet Type	Field Strength	Costs	Advantages	Disadvantages
Resistive	up to 0.15T	initially $100K or less, but power costs are high.	fewer site restrictions; possibly less down time.	lower field strengths; less spatial resolution.
Superconductive	0.15T or more	$200K or more.	better soft tissue contrast and resolution.	increased fringe fields; dependence on super-conducting technology.
Permanent	up to 0.3T	$150K or more, depending on field strength; operational costs minimal.	almost no fringe fields; minimal power and coolant; dependable operation.	weight; uniformity of field.

resistance conceivably could damage the magnet. Most superconducting magnets are protected against damage to the magnet during a quench. Even if no permanent damage occurs, several hours may be required to reestablish the superconducting condition once a quench has occurred.

Permanent units operate without extensive requirements for either electrical power or liquid helium coolant, and they are essentially free from mechanical failure. However, they are subject to resolution losses associated with nonuniformities in the magnetic field, and to problems associated with extraction of a metal object, should one become captured between the pole pieces. In one permanent magnet system, the developer has devised a clever method to tune the magnetic field to improve its uniformity. With one commercial unit employing a permanent magnet, the weight of the system (100 tons) could be a disadvantage under certain circumstances.

Small steel objects can produce significant image artifacts if they are near the region of the body being scanned (**Figure 4-2**). Dental fillings usually are nonmagnetic and do not cause artifacts, although gold fillings sometimes introduce minor distortions. Orthopedic implants usually are made from a nonmagnetic chromium-cobalt alloy and do not degrade the image. Surgical clips are stainless steel and usually have no significant magnetic properties; however, some clips do introduce slight distortions, perhaps because variations in the manufacturing process can produce microscopic regions of magnetism within the clips. Some aneurysm clips experience a torque when in the main field, and this may be hazardous enough to exclude some patients from MR examination.

For easy insertion and removal of the patient and examination table, the magnet should provide an aperture of at least 1 meter in diameter.

Magnetic Gradient

The magnetic gradient subsystem is necessary to provide a magnetic field profile so that the origin of the MR signal within the patient can be spatially decoded. Typically three sets of coils are used to produce magnetic gradients along the three dimensions of the imaging volume. To produce a gradient along the z-axis (the axis parallel to the direction of the applied magnetic field), only two coils are required (**Figure 4-3**). An electric current circulating in each coil produces an axial magnetic field that adds to the static magnetic field at one end of the coil and subtracts from it at the other end. In this manner, a gradient in the magnetic field strength is created along the longitudinal axis of the patient. This gradient permits selection of slices of tissue for transverse images.

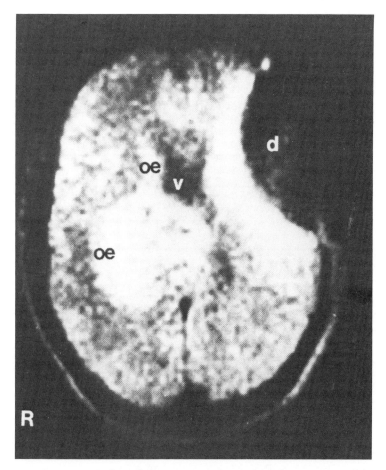

Figure 4-2. Image artifact from magnetic material. SE image showing a meningioma of the falx and its surrounding edema, **oe**, near the ventricles, **v**. The large image defect, **d**, is from magnetic field distortion around an iron splinter in the subcutaneous tissue of the scalp.

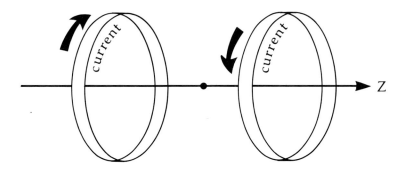

Figure 4-3. Configuration of the z-gradient coils. The coils create a gradient of magnetic field strength increasing from left to right in the direction of the primary magnetic field (indicated as the **z** axis).

To produce gradients in the transverse dimensions (i.e. in the x and y dimensions) of the patient, an additional, more complex configuration of coils is required. A representative configuration of coils to produce x and y gradients is described in **Figure 4-4**. By changing the magnitude and direction of current in these coils, gradients can be produced in any desired orientation within the x-y plane.

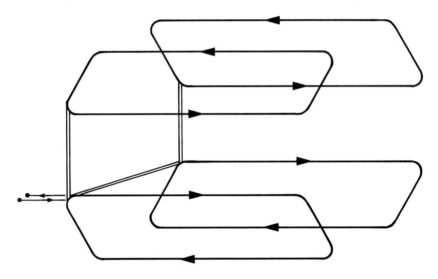

Figure 4-4. Representative configuration of coils to produce x and y gradients in magnetic field intensity for the purpose of obtaining spatially discrete MR information. (Reprinted with permission from Fullerton GD: Basic concepts of NMR imaging. Mag. Res. May 1, 1982, 39-53.)

Radiofrequency Equipment

The radiofrequency equipment consists essentially of a radio transmitter, power amplifier, transmitting and receiving coil(s), preamplifier and receivers. The electronic components in this subsystem are similar to those encountered in broadcast radio. The transmitter and receiver coil(s), on the other hand, are designed specifically for efficient transfer of radiofrequency energy into and out of the human body. For whole body imaging, two basic approaches to coil design have been followed. One approach is a solenoid coil configuration surrounding the patient that is used principally with permanent magnetic systems. The other is a set of saddle-shaped coils (Golay coils) primarily positioned alongside the patient; this approach is used with resistive and superconductive systems (1). In addition, surface coils are used to obtain low-noise images of small regions of the body. Surface coils for imaging the orbit and the breast have been reported, and others are under development. Improvement in the design of each of the coil configurations described above is a continuing effort in the search for ways to improve the signal-to-noise ratio in MR imaging.

Computer, Data Storage, and Display Unit

The radiofrequency energy emitted from the patient during an MR examination induces electronic signals in the receiver coil. These signals are transmitted to analog-digital convertors (ADCs) where they are converted into digital signals for processing by a computer. In the computer, the digital signals are used in a reconstruction algorithm to yield a matrix of numbers that can be displayed as a gray-scale of color image. Processes for the computation and display of MR data are similar to those used in computed tomography, and the reader is referred to descriptive texts in computed tomography for their explanation (2, 3).

During an MR examination, the patient is positioned inside the magnet bore and surrounded by several coils as depicted in **Figure 4-5**. The coils are hidden from view by cover plates (**Figure 4-6**), and the patient hears only the faint whine of electric current circulating in the coils and frequent, rather noisy sounds as the magnetic gradients are switched from one orientation to the next.

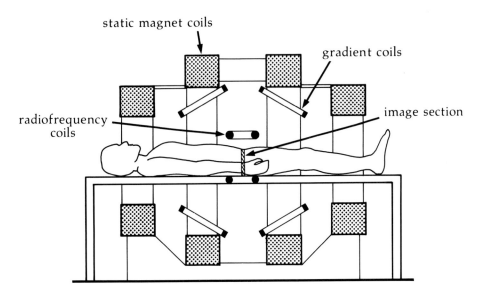

Figure 4-5. Diagram of a representative resistive-type whole body MR imaging unit.

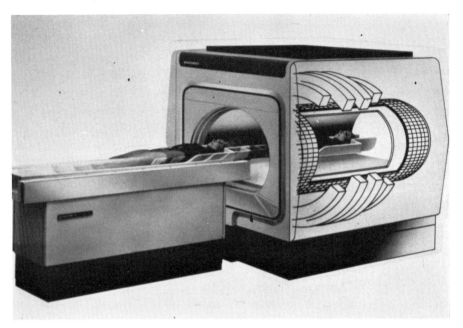

Figure 4-6. Cutaway drawing of a representative MR imaging unit.

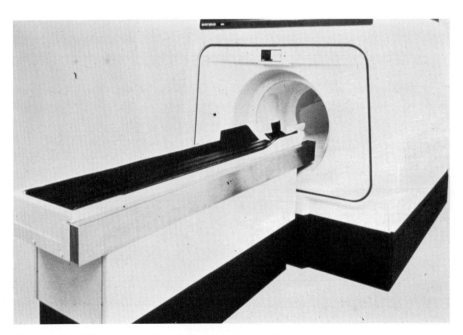

Figure 4-7. Representative MR imaging unit.

References

1. Fullerton, G.D.: Basic concepts of NMR imaging. Mag. Res. May 1: 39-53, 1982.
2. Newton, T.H., and Potts, G.D., (eds.): *Radiology of the Skull and Brain, Vol. 5: Technical Aspects of Computed Tomography.* St. Louis: 1981, C.V. Mosby, Co.
3. Hendee, W.R.: *The Physical Principles of Computed Tomography.* Boston: 1983, Little, Brown and Co.

Chapter 5
Site Selection

An MR unit, and the environment in which it is located, are mutually interactive. That is, the unit influences the environment, and the environment in turn can affect the operation of the unit. This interactive framework must be accommodated in the design of an MR facility if the unit is to produce images of highest quality in a dependable fashion. Hence, the location and design of the facility are among the more important tasks associated with the installation of an MR unit.

Magnetic Field Zones

The static magnetic field employed in MR is most intense in the core of the magnet where the patient is positioned for examination. With resistive and superconductive (but not permanent magnet units), less intense magnetic fields (1/100 to 1/1000 of core intensity) extend in all directions from the MR unit for distances of many meters. These fringe magnetic fields can affect the operation of several types of electronic devices, including photomultiplier tubes, image intensifiers, and demand-type cardiac pacemakers when they are present near an MR unit.

Fringe magnetic fields around an MR unit are often separated into various zones, as illustrated in Table 5 (1).

Table 5
The magnetic field intensity associated with various zones around an MR unit.

Zone	Intensity [gauss]
1	>15
2	5-15
3	2-5

In the more intense fringe fields of zone 1, a variety of magnetically induced events may occur. For example, there is evidence that the operation of certain types of cardiac pacemakers may be affected in the presence of magnetic fields of relatively low intensity. Although the effects may be uneventful for the average pacemaker patient over a limited time period, they could conceivably have a deleterious effect if exposure were continued over an extended period. Information stored on magnetic tape or disk could be erased if the component were brought into zone 1. Similarly, information on the magnetic strip of personal credit cards can be erased in zone 1. In the same zone, small magnetic objects like screwdrivers, pocket knives, etc., can become flying missiles, presenting serious hazards to patients and operating personnel. To avoid these problems, a screening program should be established to prevent individuals from carrying loose metallic objects into the area immediately surrounding the MR unit. For distances extending into zone 2 and even zone 3, electronic instruments may exhibit erratic behavior because of the influence of stray magnetic fields. One of the principal advantages of an MR unit employing a permanent magnet is the absence of fringe magnetic fields.

The operation of an MR unit may be affected rather severely by large masses of magnetizable materials (usually iron) in the vicinity of the unit. These materials can alter the homogeneity of the applied magnetic field and produce distortion in the resulting images. If the magnetizable materials are stationary (e.g., steel beams used for structural support or iron pipes positioned below grade), they can be compensated for by tuning small gradient coils in the MR unit. This process is termed "shimming." A greater problem is created if the masses of magnetizable materials are moving (e.g., elevators, trucks, etc.). There is essentially no fail-safe method to compensate for the effects of moving structures; the best way to prevent their influence on the MR image is to locate the unit far away from any larger moving masses of iron or other magnetizable material. For some MR units of higher field strength, a separate building to house the unit is often recommended.

It is important to recognize that the fringe fields extend not only laterally but also vertically from the MR unit. Hence, planning an MR site requires consideration of the interaction between the unit and its environment in three dimensions. Shown in **Figure 5-1** and **5-2** are the lateral and vertical dimensions of the fringe magnetic fields for a 0.5T superconductive MR system.

As the intensity of the primary magnetic field increases, the fringe fields extend farther from the MR unit. For example, the fields characterizing zone 3 might extend about 9 meters from a 0.15T MR unit; for a 1.5T system, zone 3 extends for a distance of 20 meters or so.

One of the difficulties of MR installations is that experience with them is so limited. As more installations are completed, some of the present concerns may be diminished; of course, others may arise.

Utilities Requirements

Most MR units have certain utilities requirements that must be satisfied to ensure proper operation. For example, heat from the power

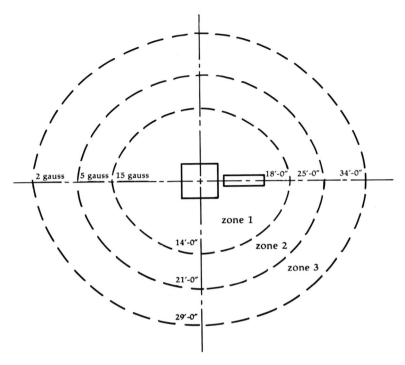

Figure 5-1. Lateral fringe magnetic fields from a 0.5T MR unit. (Courtesy of Technicare Corporation.)

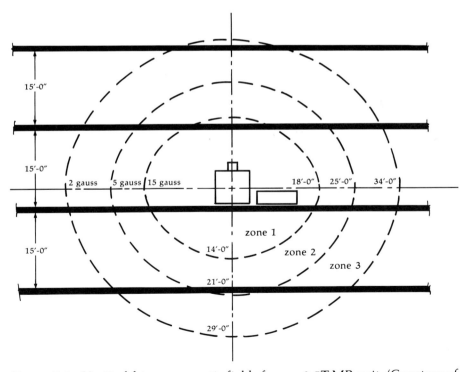

Figure 5-2. Vertical fringe magnetic fields from a 0.5T MR unit. (Courtesy of Technicare Corporation.)

supply of a resistive magnet unit is usually dissipated by circulating chilled water through the power supply. With a resistive unit, large amounts of heat must also be removed from the magnet itself by the same process; any spatial or temporal fluctuations in temperature of the magnet caused by heat build-up can create magnetic field nonuniformities that lead to distortion in the image. In general, an MR unit will perform properly only if the magnetic field is uniform to within a few parts per million.

A superconductive magnet is cooled with liquid helium and nitrogen. Proper air circulation and venting must be maintained in the room where these materials are stored to prevent accumulation of gaseous helium and nitrogen. A vent to release boil-off gases from the magnet itself is also desirable in most installations.

An MR unit employing a permanent magnet has no cooling requirements for either a magnet power supply or the magnet itself. In general, cooling of radiant coils and electronic instrumentation in a permanent magnet system can be provided by circulating air.

An MR unit will have specifications for the electrical power utilized during operation. For resistive and superconductive units, the electrical power should be supplied by a dedicated power line. A resistive MR system is by far the largest consumer of electrical energy. A superconductive system of much greater field strength will consume considerably less electricity because of the superconducting nature of its magnet. Power requirements for a permanent magnet unit are related only to the operation of ancillary coils and electronic instrumentation. In most situations it is impractical to connect an MR unit to a source of emergency power; in the event of power failure, the transition to emergency power is usually too slow to preserve the examination being conducted.

Ambient Conditions

Requirements for the control of temperature, humidity, and particulate matter in the air around an MR unit are not unlike those for other types of sophisticated electronic equipment. These requirements should be denoted by the vendor well in advance of installation of the unit. A temperature alarm should be installed in the computer room to reveal temperature fluctuations outside the operating range of the equipment.

Space

The space required for an MR unit includes the imaging room where patients are examined, a control room for operation of the unit, a computer room with closely controlled temperature, humidity, and air conditioning, and a small room for the storage of cryogens for a superconducting unit. Additional rooms may be desired for patient

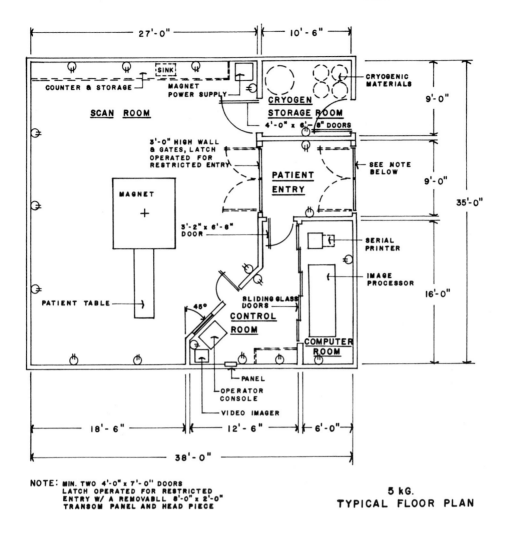

Figure 5-3. A representative facility layout for a 0.5T superconductive MR unit. (Courtesy of Technicare Corporation.)

preparation and for the interpretation and discussion of patient examinations. The patient preparation room can also serve as a dedicated life-support room for rapid patient transfer in the event of a medical emergency. In most cases, the physical layout for an MR facility resembles that for a computed tomographic unit, except that the imaging room may be somewhat larger. The actual size of the imaging room depends in part on the field strength of the unit.

In constructing an MR facility, every effort should be made to utilize nonmagnetic materials whenever possible. For example, steel beams or pipe should not be used if they are at all avoidable. Likewise, magnetic light fixtures and metallic ceiling and floor grids should not be used.

Some superconducting MR units require a rather high ceiling (e.g., 4 meters) to permit access to the magnet for replenishment of liquid helium and nitrogen. Occasionally this requirement presents some difficulty when an existing room is to be remodeled into an MR facility.

The radiofrequency (rf) signals emanating from the body during an MR examination are very weak and easily lost in the milieu of rf background. To reduce background noise, most manufacturers recommend the installation of an rf shield around the imaging room. This shield usually is copper mesh or plate fastened to all walls, floor, and ceiling of the room. It is important that no open areas in the copper cladding occur at interfaces in the rf shield along the walls, floor, and ceiling. It is also important that fluorescent light fixtures not be used in the facility; they are a major contribution to the rf background.

The magnets in an MR unit may weigh anywhere from 5 to 100 tons, depending on the type of unit and its field strength. This weight can create difficult floor loading problems, especially if the unit is to be placed above grade in an existing facility. Resistive and permanent magnets can be separated into parts for transport to the installation site; however, a superconductive magnet must remain intact once it is assembled. Access into the site for such a unit can be a challenge. A representative facility layout for a 0.5T superconductive MR unit is shown in **Figure 5-3.**

Reference

1. Technicare Corporation: NMR Imaging: 3.0 and 5.0 KGauss Systems Planning Guide, 1982.

Chapter 6
Relaxation in Normal and Diseased Tissues

Introduction

In a magnetic resonance image, the appearance of a particular tissue is determined primarily by the magnetic properties of hydrogen. Hydrogen atoms are present in water and in virtually every other compound in the body, including proteins, lipids, and nucleic acids. In an imaged region, all the hydrogen protons may be affected by rf pulses and potentially can add to the image; in fact, however, many of the protons offer no significant image contribution. In a solid, for example, the molecular structure is rigid, protons have fixed neighbors, and spin-spin relaxation times are reduced to a few microseconds. These protons experience complete spin-spin relaxation before the imaging unit begins to receive a signal from the tissue. Hence, these protons are "MR-silent." Even equipment designed to receive an MR signal immediately following an rf pulse generally cannot detect a signal from these protons, because their extremely short T_2 decreases the signal intensity to a level below detectability. For tissues in a magnetic resonance image, there is no significant signal contribution from protons in solid-like constituents such as DNA, RNA, or proteins.

In a proton magnetic resonance image, the signal is derived primarily from tissue water and secondarily from lipids. Hence, the measured T_1 and T_2 values of a particular tissue largely reflect the T_1 and T_2 values of the water content of the tissue. Water is a molecule with an asymmetric charge distribution that results in the formation of hydrogen bonds with adjacent molecules. These hydrogen bonds are often formed with the chemical side groups of macromolecules, particularly the carboxyl and amine side groups of proteins. These bonds help stabilize the three-dimensional structure of cell membranes and proteins and aid in maintaining enzymes in their active configuration. The bonding of water to macromolecules substantially reduces the thermal tumbling of water molecules, slowing them down and restricting them to certain types of motion. This restricted motion significantly alters the T_1 and T_2 values of tissue water compared to pure water.

65

Theories of Water Relaxation

Spin-spin and spin-lattice relaxation are a result of magnetic field fluctuations arising from the motion of protons and molecules in the surrounding lattice. The motion of protons produced by the rotational, translational, and vibrational movement of molecules containing hydrogen is a major source of these magnetic field fluctuations. The first general theory describing the relationships among T_1, T_2, and molecular motion was published in 1948 (1). A quantity important in these relationships is the diffusional or translational correlation time (t_c), a measurable quantity that represents the average time a molecule spends at one point in space before changing to a new location. For a typical molecule in pure water, t_c is about 10^{-12} second and its motion has frequency components from 0 to 10^{12} Hz (2). A plot of the intensity of motion as a function of frequency assumes different shapes for different values of t_c. The plot is rather broad and flat for pure water (**Figure 6-1**), reflecting the wide range of frequencies of about equal intensities present in the motion of pure water molecules. In ice, molecular motion is rather restricted because the molecules are bound together in a rigid three-dimensional structure. In ice the t_c is about 10^{-6} second, and the range of motional frequencies of a water molecule varies from 0 to 10^6 Hz. For water molecules in ice, a plot of motion

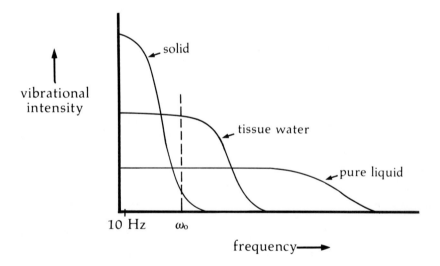

Figure 6-1. Motion (translation, rotation, and vibration). Intensity as a function of frequency for solid water (ice), tissue water, and for pure liquid water. The area under each curve is identical. Higher intensity at the Larmor frequency (ω_o) stimulates T_1 and T_2 while higher intensity at lower frequencies (about 10 Hz) stimulates T_2 but not T_1. The intensity at ω_o is greater for tissue water than for either solid or pure liquid, and so T_1 is reduced. The intensity at 10 Hz is intermediate for tissue water compared to solid and pure liquid and therefore its T_2 is also intermediate.

intensity versus frequency is taller and narrower compared to that for liquid water. The shape of this plot reveals a greater intensity of low-frequency motion and a lower intensity of high-frequency motion in ice compared to liquid water. Water molecules bound to tissue constituents have a t_c of about 10^{-8} second, with considerable intensity at moderately high frequencies and reduced intensity at low frequencies.

The values of T_1 and T_2 are determined largely by the intensity of molecular motion at two specific frequencies. Spin-lattice and spin-spin relaxation are both stimulated (i.e., T_1 and T_2 are shortened) by greater intensity of motion at the Larmor frequency (about 5×10^5 - 5×10^6 Hz for current imaging systems). Spin-lattice relaxation is also stimulated by low-frequency components (about 10 Hz) (3). T_1 for tissue water is less than T_1 for either ice or pure water because intensity of motion (primarily vibrational) at the Larmor frequency is greater in tissue water (Table 6). The T_2 value for tissue water is between the T_2 values for ice and pure water because the vibrational intensity of tissue water has an intermediate value at low frequencies.

Table 6

Vibrational intensity at the Larmor frequency and at low frequencies, and the relaxation constants T_1 and T_2 in ice, tissue water, and liquid water.

	Vibrational Intensity at the Larmor Frequency	T_1	Vibrational Intensity at Low Frequency	T_2
Ice	Low	Long	High	Short
Tissue Water	Moderate	Intermediate	Moderate	Intermediate
Liquid Water	Low	Long	Low	Long

The general theory relating T_1 and T_2 dependence to the degree of molecular motion applies directly to homogeneous systems. Several attempts have been made to develop a model that explains the observed NMR properties of tissue by considering the inhomogeneity of tissue. A satisfactory model should estimate T_1 and T_2 accurately and should predict the self-diffusion coefficient (D), where D is related to the time required for two neighboring water molecules to exchange places. NMR measurements show that, compared to pure water: T_1 of tissue water is less by a factor of 10; T_2 is less by a factor of 100; and D is less by a factor of 4 to 7 (4).

The simplest and most popular model of tissue water is that proposed by Zimmerman and Brittin (5). In this model, two phases of water exist around macromolecules. One phase is tightly bound to macromolecules and represents the water of hydration. This water phase has restricted motion ($t_c \simeq 10^{-8}$ second), extends for only a very short distance from macromolecular surfaces, and accounts for less than 5% of the total water. In this model more than 95% of cell water is essentially free of any influence from macromolecules. This water has the properties of water in a bulk aqueous solution with a t_c of about 10^{-12} second. Water molecules in the two phases exchange with each other, and the item that characterizes the exchange process determines the overall relaxation behavior of the sample. In general, biological systems are described by a "fast exchange" model in which the time required for a water molecule to exchange between the phases is shorter than the relaxation times in either phase. The resulting relaxation behavior is dominated by the properties of the much smaller, tightly bound water fraction and can be described by a single exponential equation. Small fluctuations in the interactions between the tightly bound phase and biological macromolecules have a major impact on the apparent relaxation times. In the Zimmerman-Brittin model the bulk of intracellular water plays no significant role in the values of T_1 and T_2.

Some investigators have found the two-phase model inadequate to explain the results of their experiments. A variety of other models have been proposed, including three phase exchange models (6). Some authors emphasize the importance of cross-relaxation, a mechanism in which proton transfer from bulk water to bound water and then to macromolecules provides an additional relaxation mechanism (6). Objections to the fast exchange model are that it does not accurately predict T_1 and T_2 values simultaneously (7), and that it does not accurately predict observed values for D (2). Some have tried to improve the fast exchange model by adding molecules to the model that serve as barriers to the free diffusion of water.

Models for bound (i.e., intracellular) water may be separated into two principal categories. Most models follow the Zimmerman-Brittin concept with or without modification. Others incorporate the hypothesis that a large fraction of intracellular water, much greater than the 5% proposed by Zimmerman-Brittin, has reduced motion. These theories assert that the influence of a macromolecule may extend a significant distance from the surface of the macromolecule. This approach presupposes that most cell water has properties that are significantly different from those of dilute aqueous solutions, consistent with the apparent reduction of D in biological systems.

Confusion about the relaxation behavior of cell water appears to be the result of two oversimplifications. First, data have been interpreted within the confines of a model that probably oversimplifies complex interactions. Second, NMR measurements are obtained over a time scale of milliseconds and represent an averaging of much more rapid processes (7). Further understanding of the relaxation of cell water may require experiments with modalities that measure events on a much shorter time scale than those accessible by NMR. Despite confusion about details, interactions between water and intracellular macromolecules do influence the T_1 and T_2 values of a tissue in a significant manner. The next section describes a number of structural variations known to occur in diseased tissues that could affect the T_1 and T_2 values in these tissues.

Microscopic and Molecular Alterations in Diseased Tissues

As revealed by electron microscopy, the ultrastructure of living cells is extremely complex (**Figure 6-2**). Cells have a three-dimensional lattice of extremely thin filaments called microtrabeculae that are 100 to 200 Å in diameter and 500 to 2000 Å apart (4, 8). The microtrabecular lattice is involved in many cell functions. Ribosomes that mediate protein synthesis are anchored at lattice intersections, and the lattice appears to play an important role in organizing the production of proteins (9). Microtrabeculae are also thought to anchor enzymes, to help organize metabolic pathways (4), to assist in the organization of genetic material in the nucleus during cell division, and to control cell shape and movement (9).

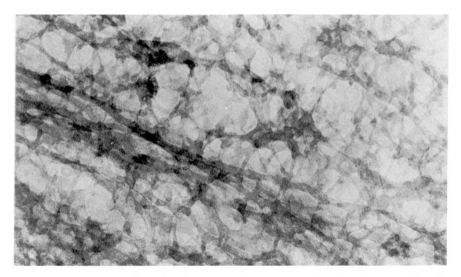

Figure 6-2. Microtrabecular lattice. The microtrabecular lattice fills the cytoplasm and helps organize a variety of cell functions. It also provides a large surface area for water-protein interactions. Individual filaments are about 6 x 10^{-6}mm thick. (Courtesy of Dr. Keith Porter.)

The microtrabecular structure divides the cytoplasm into a multitude of tiny interconnecting pockets and hence has a large surface area.

In diseased cells, changes in the microtrabeculae may exert significant effects on the interactions between water and macromolecules. These interactions should influence the values of T_1 and T_2. Immunofluorescent light microscopy of human breast cancer cells reveals a correlation between cell growth rates and disorganization or loss of the microtrabecular structure (10) (**Figure 6-3**). These studies suggest that T_1 and T_2 changes in cancer may arise, at least in part, from changes in water-microtrabecular interactions (10).

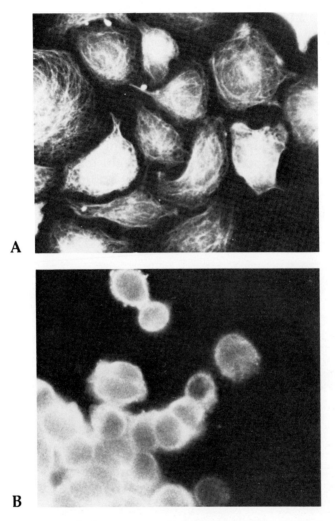

Figure 6-3. Microtubular structure in malignant cells. Immunofluorescence antibody staining for tubulin protein (thought to represent the microtubular structure) in human breast cancer cells shows that the protein is partly preserved in moderate growing cells, **A**, but lost in fast-growing cells, **B**. Loss of these fine cytoplasmic structures may lead to less structured cell water, decreased t_c, and prolonged relaxation. (Reprinted with permission from Beall, P.T., and others: Microtubule complexes correlated with growth rate and water proton relaxation times in human breast cancer cells. Cancer Res. 42:4124-4130, 1982.)

Some authors have detected a gradual increase in T_1 and T_2 as cells progress from normal through neoplastic to a fully malignant state (11). In general, although there are exceptions, tumors appear to exhibit prolonged T_1 and T_2 relaxation times compared to preneoplastic or benign lesions. A prominent feature of malignant cells is disorganization of the nucleus; this disorganization may reflect abnormal nuclear water-macromolecular interactions and contribute to the prolonged values of T_1 and T_2 observed for tumors.

In some cases, observed T_1 and T_2 changes may reflect an increase in intercellular water (edema). Several authors have identified a direct correlation between the increased water content of tissues and prolonged relaxation times accompanying a variety of disease states (6, 12). Edema often develops around regions of tissue injury and tumors because of the extravasation of protein-rich fluid from blood vessels.

Distinction between the separate contributions of intracellular and intercellular water relaxation to the overall relaxation characteristics of a tissue is difficult. Estimates of the intercellular fluid volume by electron microscopy reveal that 20% of the fluid is intercellular in normal white matter, and that this fraction may increase to 40% in edema induced by freezing a small portion of the cerebral cortex in animals (13, 14). In this particular study, the amount of intracellular water changed very little, and the relaxation data could be explained solely by changes in the relaxation of intercellular water, according to a two-fraction fast exchange model where the two fractions are bulk intercellular water and water bound to the outer surface of myelin sheaths. Relaxation changes might also occur because cell debris and cell proteins released into intercellular spaces by damaged cells alter the state of intercellular water and produce changes in the relaxation of this fluid (15).

The earliest change observed in ischemia is a decrease in cellular ATP. This change can be detected quickly by ^{31}P NMR spectroscopy; changes in proton images are observed somewhat later (16). The earliest observed structural changes in ischemia are clumping of nuclear chromatin and the disappearance of mitochondrial granules. These changes are followed by swelling of other microscopic structures, distortion of the cell membrane, and increasing distortion and swelling of mitochondria (16). All of these changes occur within 15 minutes after the onset of ischemia. The clumping of chromatin and the swelling of mitochondria probably reflect changes in water-macromolecular interactions. However, these early intracellular effects do not necessarily contribute significantly to early changes in the macroscopic appearance of ischemic tissue. Changes in NMR images that reflect alterations in T_1 and T_2 are not generally observed earlier than 90 minutes following the onset of ischemia (17). Following stroke, the appearance of ischemic changes observed by NMR parallels the increases in the water content of the affected tissue (17, 18).

71

Lipid Relaxation

Triglycerides are long-chain lipid molecules that tumble and twist in space because of thermal motion. The t_c of this motion is similar to the t_c value for cell water. A magnetic resonance signal from the protons in triglycerides can be detected with an MR unit. Adipose tissue is rich in triglycerides; subcutaneous fat, fat around abdominal organs, and fat in bone marrow are all clearly visible in magnetic resonance images.

A possible role has been identified for lipid proteins in the relaxation characteristics of diseased tissues. Fossel has recently obtained proton chemical shift data from a human breast cancer in a high-field NMR spectrometer (19). These data permitted the separation of the relaxation behaviors of tissue water and lipid protons and led to detection of a significant prolongation of the T_1 of lipid protons in the tumor compared to normal tissue. Other investigations have separated the relaxation of lipid from the relaxation of water protons in human breast cancers and have also found that tumor water relaxation is unchanged, suggesting that the tumor lipid protons alone may be responsible for prolonged relaxation times (20).

Conclusion

There are several ways in which disease processes can alter the NMR relaxation properties of tissues. Although interactions between intracellular water and macromolecules have been studied extensively, there is no general agreement on the amount of intracellular water which has restricted motion. Resolution of this question is important for cell physiologists, cell biologists, and NMR experimenters; if a major portion of intracellular water is ordered, then many beliefs about cell function and metabolism, as well as the two-fraction fast exchange model of relaxation, are incorrect. The relaxation characteristics of normal body tissues are even more complex. The state of organization of nuclear material, water-microtrabecular and other water-macromolecular interactions, increased amount of intercellular water and macromolecules and changes in their interactions, changes in lipid relaxation, and possibly other mechanisms may all contribute to the macroscopic NMR behavior of body tissues. The significant components may be different for acute and chronic stages of the same disease. Considerable research will be necessary before the significance of pathology revealed by MR can be unraveled.

References

1. Bloembergen, N., Purcell, E.M., and Pound R.V.: Relaxation effects in nuclear magnetic resonance absorption. Phys. Rev. 73:679-712, 1948.

2. Farrar, T.C. and Becker, E.D.: *Pulse and Fourier Transform NMR.* New York: 1971, Academic Press, Inc.

3. Mathur-DeVrie R.: The NMR studies of water in biological systems. Prog. Biophys. Mol. 35:103-134, 1979.

4. Clegg, J.S.: Properties and metabolism of the aqueous cytoplasm and its boundaries. Am. J. Physiol. In press.

5. Zimmerman, J.R., and Brittin, W.E.: Nuclear magnetic resonance studies in multiple phase systems: lifetime of a water molecule in an absorbing phase on silica gel. J. Phys. Chem. 61:1328-1333, 1957.

6. Ratkovic, S.: NMR studies of water in biological system at different levels of their organization. Scientia Yugoslavica 7:19-64, 1981.

7. Beall, P.T.: States of water in biological systems. Cryobiology 20:324-334, 1983.

8. Porter, K.R., and others: The distribution of water in the cytoplasm. 40th Annual Proc. Elec. Micros. Soc. Amer., 1982, 4-7.

9. Porter, K.R., and Tucker, J.B.: The ground substance of the living cell. Sci. Amer. 244:56-67, 1981.

10. Beall, P.T., and others: Microtubule complexes correlated with growth rate and water proton relaxation times in human breast cancer cells. Canc. Res. 42:4124-4130, 1982.

11. Beall, P.T., and others: Distinction of normal, preoplastic and neoplastic mouse mammary primary cell cultures by water nuclear magnetic resonance relaxation times. J. Nat. Canc. Inst. 64:335-338, 1980.

12. Saryan, L.A., and others: Nuclear magnetic resonance studies of cancer, IV. Correlation of water content with tissue relaxation times. J. Nat. Canc. Inst. 52:599-602, 1974.

13. Bakay, L., and others: Nuclear magnetic resonance studies in normal and edematous brain tissue. Exp. Brain Res. 23:241-248, 1975.

14. Lee, J.C., and Bakay, L.: Ultrastructural changes in the edematous central nervous system, II. Cold induced edema. Arch. Neurol. 14:36-49, 1966.

15. Stark, D.D., and others: Nuclear magnetic resonance imaging of experimentally induced liver disease. Radiology 148:743-751, 1983.

16. Trump, B.F., and others: Recent studies on the pathophysiology of ischemic cell injury. Beitr. Path. Bd. 158:363-388, 1976.

17. Buonanno, F.S., and others: Proton NMR imaging in ischemic infarction. Stroke 14:178-184, 1983.

18. Spetzler, R.F., and others: Acute NMR changes during MCA occlusion; a preliminary study in primates. Stroke 14:185-191, 1983.

19. Fossel, E.T.: Physiologic studies. In: Proc. 1st Ann. Mtg. Soc. Mag. Reson. Med., Boston, August 1982.

20. Bovee, W.M., and others: Nuclear magnetic resonance and detection of human breast tumors. J. Nat. Canc. Inst. 61:53-55, 1978.

Chapter 7
Magnetic Resonance Imaging of the Central Nervous System

Introduction

MR image quality has improved phenomenally in a very few years. The first high-quality images of the head were produced in 1981 (1), and the first clinical trial was published in 1982 (2). In the 18 months following that publication, over one hundred papers on the clinical applications of MR images were published. Much of the early clinical work has been a mixture of identifying normal appearances, establishing basic signs in various diseases, and comparing MR to other techniques (3). Many universities have purchased MR units, and many others will soon do so. Several thousand patients have been examined, and the number is increasing rapidly. Although it may be a few years before the ultimate contribution of MR to medical imaging is known, it appears already that MR will have a major impact, particularly in dealing with the central nervous system.

MR has several advantages over other imaging modalities. Inversion recovery images provide superb contrast between gray and white matter. Lesion localization is precise and mass effects are easy to detect. There are no significant artifacts at the base of the skull, in the posterior fossa, at the skull apex, and around the jaw. Dental fillings and most surgical clips do not significantly degrade the MR image. Transverse, sagittal, and coronal sections may all be made (sequentially in multislice reconstruction, simultaneously in volume reconstruction) without reformatting and without moving the patient. Coronal and sagittal sections are helpful in evaluating longitudinal structures such as the spine and brain stem and in demonstrating the cranial-caudal extent of lesions and the displacement and/or infiltration of neighboring structures. They may be used at the skull apex, skull base, and near the roof of the orbit to avoid partial volume effects found in transverse images of these regions. T_1 and T_2 may change by 100% or more in diseased tissue, while x-ray attenuation changes only a few percent. Hence, MR often reveals a disease earlier and shows the full extent of the disease more faithfully than modalities based on transmitted x rays. Its lack of ionizing radiation may make it more acceptable than CT in some pediatric cases, particularly when frequent imaging is required. Considerable information can be obtained without the use of contrast agents, and patients who are hypersensitive to iodine can be examined safely. Finally, a number of pulse sequences may be used in MR, and both the interpulse delay and the repetition time may be varied widely. Contrast between a lesion and normal tissue, or between different organs, can be optimized, and blood flow can be measured or used to enhance image contrast.

MR reveals abnormalities missed by CT in a significant fraction of patients, characterizes the nature or extent of disease better in a few, and displays more lesions in many cases of multifocal disease (4). In the central nervous system, the most definitive applications of MR appear to be in demyelinating diseases such as multiple sclerosis (MS), in the posterior fossa, in patients with a focal neurological exam and a normal CT, in the spinal cord and at the craniovertebral junction, and in some tumors arising in or around the sella turcica. The specificity of MR is somewhat diminished by the current lack of contrast agents and the insensitivity of the method to calcification. For certain medical problems, images providing both T_1 and T_2 discrimination may be required for complete characterization.

Pulse Sequences

In the first clinical studies of normal anatomy and pathology in the central nervous system, inversion recovery was used extensively (2). The pulse sequence reveals brain anatomy and subtle mass effects in exquisite detail. It detects disease processes with high sensitivity through differences principally in T_1. In many cases, moderate TR/moderate TI sequences appear to provide optimum anatomic discrimination and lesion sensitivity (2). Occasionally, problems arise because most lesions have prolonged T_1 values and yield a reduced MR signal. It can be difficult to see small lesions because they blend with normal gray matter, particularly in the cerebral cortex. Lesions also may be difficult to visualize if they are adjacent to bone, which is always dark because of its low mobile proton density, or to CSF, which has low intensity in IR images because of its long T_1. The use of short rather than moderate TI intervals reverses lesion contrast and makes regions of prolonged T_1 brighter, possibly improving the detectability of lesions adjacent to bone (2).

Partial saturation sequences can also provide images with T_1 weighting. Compared to inversion recovery techniques, more pulse sequence repetitions can be obtained in a given scan time with partial saturation. The resulting increase in signal intensity of PS images compensates for their somewhat poorer T_1 contrast resolution compared to IR (5). In some cases, lesion detectability may be better with PS than with IR.

Spin-echo sequences are very versatile and may currently be the most clinically useful sequences in the CNS. Most lesions have prolonged T_2 values and are revealed with high intensity compared to brain and CSF in moderate TE images. Multiple sclerosis lesions (6), a variety of primary and metastatic tumors, cytotoxic and vasogenic edema, and various white matter diseases are readily demonstrable with a moderate TE spin-echo image. In these lesions, increased T_1 tends to decrease lesion intensity in spin-echo images; hence moderate or long TR intervals are frequently used with moderate TE parameters to increase lesion detectability for routine imaging. Once a lesion has been detected, pulse sequences can be refined to highlight the internal structure of the lesion.

Normal Anatomy

Fat in the scalp is white and outlines the skull. The inner and outer tables of the skull are black because of their low proton density. In some regions, a signal from fat in the diploic space can be seen. Fat in the orbit is also bright. The darkness of the inner table allows the surface of adjacent brain to be seen clearly. Blood vessels have dark lumens in most images because of blood flow. CSF has a long T_1 and moderate T_2 and is dark in IR, PS, and short TR/short TE spin-echo images. The ventricles, subarachnoid spaces, and basal cisterns stand out with these sequences (**Figures 7-1** and **7-2**). The sagittal plane is ideal for displaying the third and fourth ventricles, brain stem, and craniovertebral junction (**Figure 7-3**). In high-quality images, the cerebral aqueduct may be seen.

IR and PS sequences yield images with good T_1 discrimination and reveal cerebellar folia, cerebral sulci, the insular cortex, amygdala, columns of the fornix, basal ganglia, cerebellar peduncles, dentate nucleus, substantia nigra, red nucleus, optic nerves, optic chiasm, and sometimes crainial nerves near the brain stem. Small brain stem nuclei generally are not visible (7). Anatomic detail is also good in long TR/long TE SE images that accentuate the shorter T_2 and lower proton density of white matter relative to gray matter. The definition of the lateral margins of the caudate nucleus allows its area and degree of atrophy to be measured in Huntington's chorea (2). Clear delineation of the sylvian fissure provides a tool for **in vivo** anatomic study of aphasia syndromes (8).

Stroke

In most cases, stroke cannot be detected reliably with CT within the first 24 hours. Hence, CT is used over this interval only to exclude other diseases. MR is more sensitive and demonstrates the extent of stroke better than CT at all states (4). It detects lesions in about 10% of patients with a normal CT (8, 9) (**Figure 7-4**); furthermore, no strokes delineated by CT are missed with MR (8) (**Figure 7-5**).

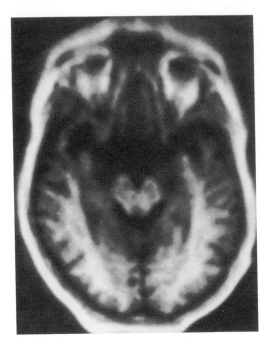

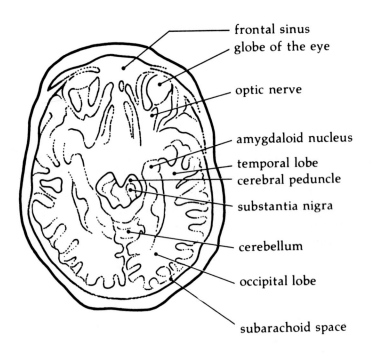

frontal sinus
globe of the eye

optic nerve

amygdaloid nucleus

temporal lobe
cerebral peduncle

substantia nigra

cerebellum

occipital lobe

subarachoid space

Figure 7-1. Normal cerebral anatomy: transverse IR. Section through the orbit and midbrain. (Reprinted with permission from Simmonds, D., and others: NMR anatomy of the brain using inversion-recovery sequences. Neuroradiology 25:113-118, 1983.)

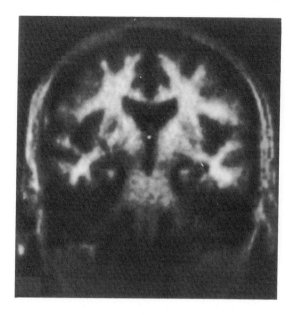

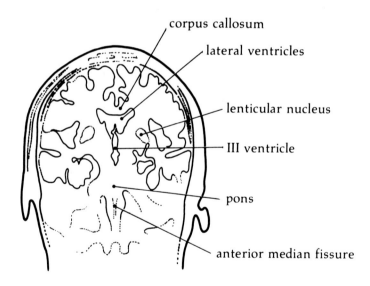

corpus callosum

lateral ventricles

lenticular nucleus

III ventricle

pons

anterior median fissure

Figure 7-2. Normal cerebral anatomy: coronal IR. (Reprinted with permission from Simmonds, D., and others: NMR anatomy of the brain using inversion-recovery sequences. Neuroradiology 25:113-118, 1983.)

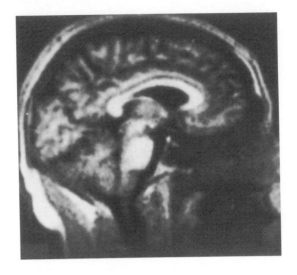

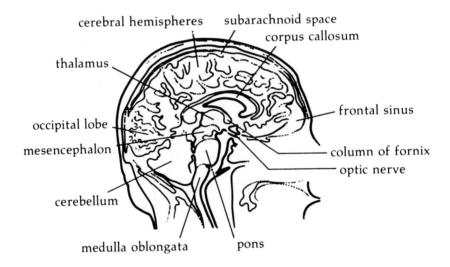

Figure 7-3. Normal cerebral anatomy: sagittal IR. (Reprinted with permission from Simmonds, D., and others: NMR anatomy of the brain using inversion-recovery sequences. Neuroradiology 25:113-118, 1983.)

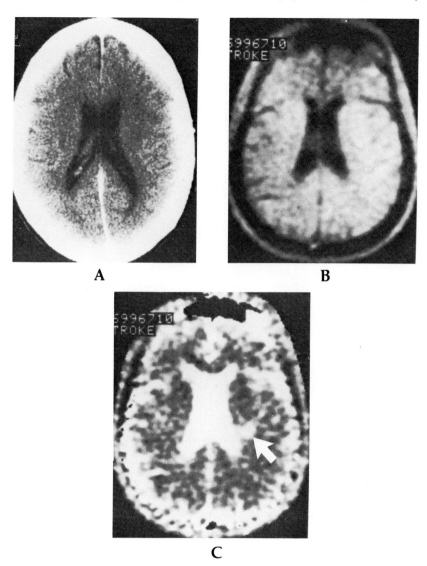

Figure 7-4. Nine-day-old stroke. A, contrast-enhanced CT. **B,** proton density. **C,** calculated T_2 images. The CT and proton density images are normal, while the calculated T_2 image reveals T_2 prolongation in a region of parietal lobe ischemia adjacent to the body of the ventricle (arrow). (Reprinted with permission from Bryn, R.M., and others: Nuclear magnetic resonance evaluation of stroke. Radiology 149:189-192, 1983.)

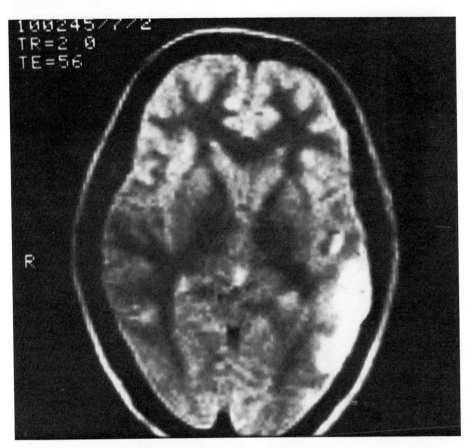

Figure 7-5. Cortical infarction: SE. This lesion could not be reliably differentiated from other conditions on the basis of T_1 and T_2 values alone, but the cortical distribution indicates its nature. (Courtesy of William G. Bradley, M.D., Ph.D.)

The exact location of a stroke is easily established, whether in the cortex, the white matter of the hemispheres, or the posterior fossa (8). Subtle mass effects that are invisible in CT images can be seen in IR scans. Lacunar infarcts are generally small and circular, as in CT, and multiple lesions frequently are seen with MR (8). Approximately 70% of clinical brain stem infarctions can be identified (2) and often have a shape corresponding to the territory of a circumferential artery. Infarctions in the posterior fossa can be visualized with the same sensitivity as in the cerebral hemispheres.

Some interesting variations in T_1 and T_2 have been observed for different types of stroke. In both acute (10) and lacunar (8) infarction, T_2 may be lengthened more than T_1. Variations in the T_1 and T_2 values of lacunar infarctions may be related to the age of individual lesions (8). Hemorrhage prolongs T_2 and shortens T_1 initially; then as the hemorrhage ages, T_1 becomes prolonged (33) (**Figure 7-6**). Areas of hemor-

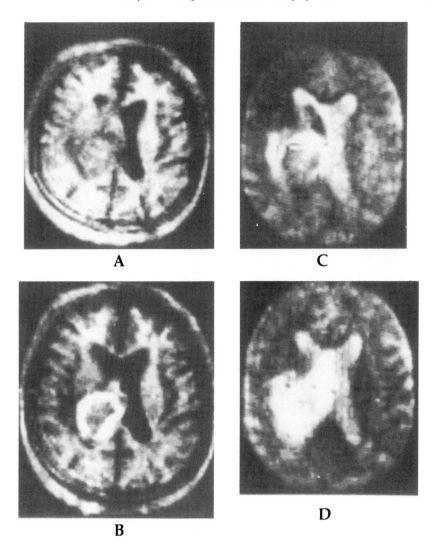

Figure 7-6. Intracerebral hemorrhage: IR and SE. A, long TR/moderate TI inversion recovery image shows that the hemorrhage has areas of increased T_1 that are imaged with low-intensity 2 days after the onset of symptoms. **B,** one week after the onset of symptoms, T_1 is shortened in some regions of the hemorrhage, producing higher intensity areas in this IR image. SE images reveal that the hemorrhage has a prolonged T_2 at 2 days, **C,** and one week, **D.** The higher intensity of the hemorrhage in **D** compared to **C** indicates further T_2 prolongation as the hemorrhage ages. (Reprinted with permission from Sipponen, J.T., and others: Nuclear magnetic resonance [NMR] imaging of intracerebral hemorrhage in the acute and resolving phases. J. Comput. Assist. Tomog. 7:954-959, 1983.)

rhagic infarction and edema may be indistinguishable in SE images because they are both displayed as high-intensity regions; however, these conditions can be differentiated in T_1 weighted sequences (4).

Surgical ligation of major cerebral vessels in animals has been used to assess the evolution of stroke. Intensity changes in the territory of the middle cerebral artery, and mild mass effects in the lateral ventricles, have been observed within 90 minutes (11). Intensity changes are usually detectable within 2 hours in major strokes (12). T_1 and T_2 increase linearly (12, 13) and reach 130 to 150% of normal values at 24 hours (13). Contrast between normal and abnormal brain apparently is maximum with moderate or long TR/long TE images and is obtained at about 24 hours following the onset of stroke (13).

Magnetic resonance images of sodium yield a strong signal from infarction and very little from normal brain, because it has a low sodium concentration (14). An infarcted region is more intense than CSF, despite similar sodium concentrations, suggesting that the sodium is more "visible" in the infarction. The signal from sodium is about 400 times weaker than that from protons, and sodium images must be obtained with magnets of high field strength. With sodium imaging, imaging times of several hours and poor spatial resolution appear to be unavoidable.

Tumors

CT is very sensitive in depicting brain tumors; however, MR appears to be even more sensitive. Occasionally CT misses tumors involving a major part of a hemisphere; these tumors are readily detectable by MR (15) because of its superb soft tissue discrimination (**Figure 7-7**). This advantage may permit the early discovery of some primary tumors, at a stage where they are still operable. MR may be useful in metastatic disease because a favorable response to chemotherapy and radiation treatment is accompanied by a decrease in T_1 (16). After treatment, an area of tumor recurrence tends to develop increased relaxation times (4, 16).

Tumors and associated edema characteristically have prolonged T_1 and T_2 values. They are easily identified (17) and can be differentiated from vascular lesions and hematomas on the basis of T_1 (18). Differentiation from inflammatory lesions and stroke is more difficult (**Figure 7-8**). The correlation among T_1, T_2 and the degree of malignancy is unknown at this time. Tumors with different cell types frequently cannot be differentiated; morphology and clinical data are both very important, as they are in CT.

Tumor characteristics such as necrosis, cyst formation, and hemorrhage often can be distinguished with MR (3); however, problems may exist in distinguishing a tumor from its surrounding edema (**Figure 7-9**) and in detecting calcification (**Figure 7-10**). Tumor T_1 and T_2 values may be either shorter or longer than edema, and pulse sequences must be tailored to maximize the contrast between them (**Figure 7-11**). In moderate TI inversion recovery images, for example, long TR intervals are necessary (8). With proper choice of pulse sequence and imaging parameters, MR may display the tumor margin better than contrast-enhanced CT (19). SE scans are more likely to identify calcium within lesions because the lesion is light and outlines the dark calcium (20). SE is also helpful in defining meningiomas adjacent to bone because most meningiomas will be displayed as a region of decreased intensity surrounded by bright CSF in long TR/long TE images.

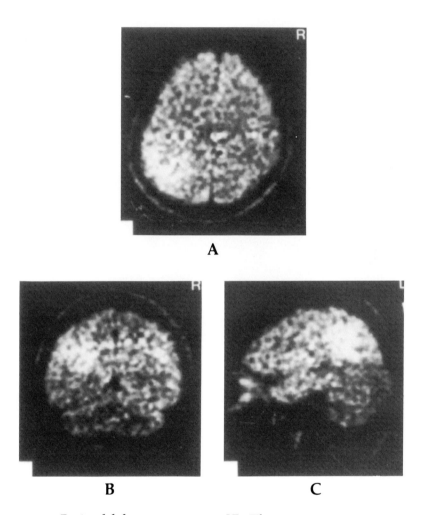

A

B   **C**

Figure 7-7. Parietal lobe astrocytoma: SE. The tumor is seen in **A**, transverse, **B**, coronal, and **C**, sagittal images as a region of increased intensity. The CT examination was normal in this patient. (Reprinted with permission from Von Einsiedel, G.H., and Loffler, W.: Nuclear magnetic resonance imaging of brain tumors unrevealed by CT. Eur. J. Radiol. 2:225-234, 1982.)

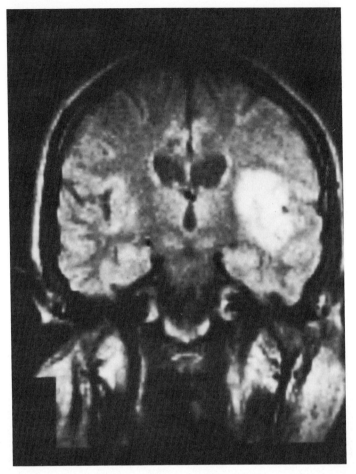

Figure 7-8. Low grade astrocytoma: SE. The lesion stands out clearly but its MR appearance is nonspecific. Inflammation, infarction, gliosis, and other conditions could present a similar picture. (Courtesy of William G. Bradley, M.D., Ph.D.)

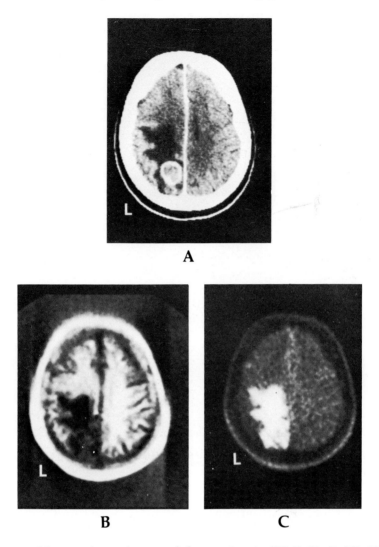

A

B   C

Figure 7-9. Metastatic carcinoma of the cervix. A, CT; **B**, IR; **C**, SE. All three images show an abnormality, but only the contrast-enhanced CT shows the metastasis separate from the surrounding edema. (Reprinted with permission from Bailes, D.R., and others: NMR imaging of the brain using spin-echo sequences. Clin. Radiol. 33:395-414, 1982.)

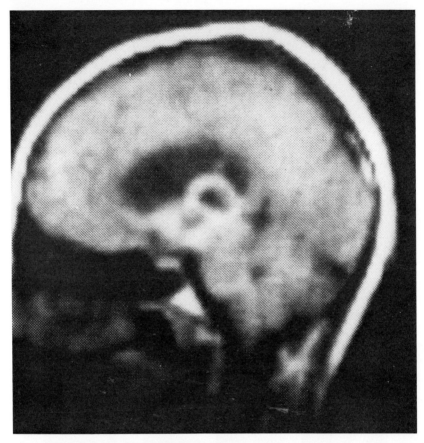

Figure 7-10. Craniopharyngioma: steady-state free precession [SSFP].
Steady-state free precession is a pulse sequencing technique in which a suc-
cession of rf pulses is applied with a short interpulse interval compared to
both T_1 and T_2. In this technique, signal intensity is a complex function of
T_1/T_2, so that the separate influences of T_1 and T_2 are difficult to distinguish.
For this reason, SSFP is infrequently used. The tumor encroaches on the
foramen of Monro. It has two lobes with low-intensity centers. Heavy peripheral calcification of this tumor is visible with CT but not with MR.
(Reprinted with permission from Hawkes, R.C., and others: The application of
NMR imaging to the evaluation of pituitary and juxtasellar tumors. Am. J.
Neuroradiol. 4:221-222, 1983.)

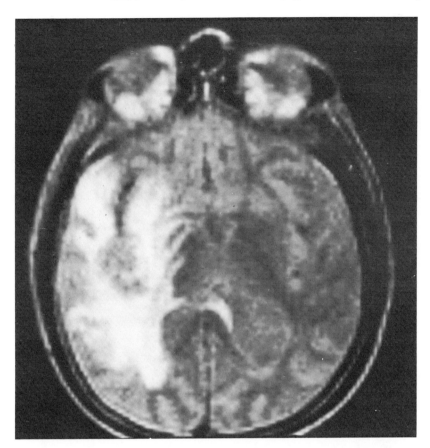

Figure 7-11. Grade III astrocytoma: short TR/moderate TE spin-echo. The tumor mass can be distinguished because the T_1 of the tumor is significantly greater than the T_1 of edema, leading to a decreased intensity for the tumor compared to the edema. (Courtesy of William G. Bradley, M.D., Ph.D.)

Sagittal images are best for evaluating the pituitary gland. The normal pituitary has the same intensity as brain and is surrounded by dark bone and CSF. Erosion of the sellar floor is not visible directly; however, bulging of the pituitary inferiorly may suggest erosion (21) (**Figure 7-12**). MR is superior to CT in evaluating extension of pituitary tumors outside the sella; the relationship of tumor to the optic tracts and invasion of adjacent structures can be observed directly (**Figure 7-13**). MR cannot always identify small adenomas because of difficulties in obtaining thin sections and because of the limited spatial resolution currently available. MR may prove helpful in identifying cystic pituitary lesions because they contrast sharply with the normal gland, while adenomas have slightly prolonged or even shortened relaxation times. Other conditions, including empty sella, have been diagnosed with MR (21). When iodinated contrast cannot be used because of severe allergy, MR gives more information than CT in suspected pituitary disease (18).

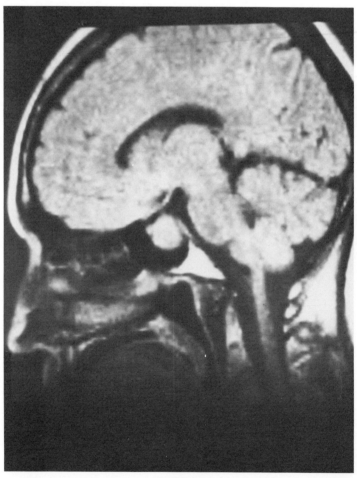

A

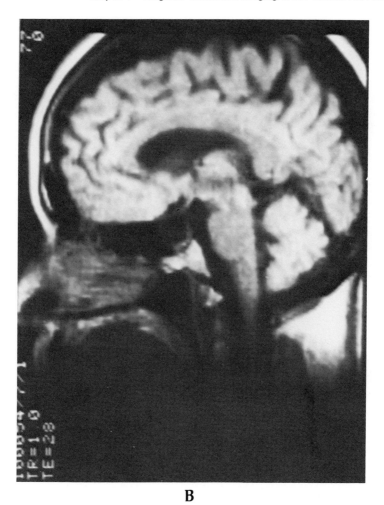

B

Figure 7-12. Pituitary adenoma and empty sella: SE. A, the normal pituitary has been replaced by an adenoma with a slightly increased intensity and greater volume than the normal gland. **B,** fluid with magnetic resonance characteristics similar to CSF fills the sella. A thin layer of normal pituitary tissue remains along with the sellar floor. (Courtesy of William G. Bradley, M.D., Ph.D.)

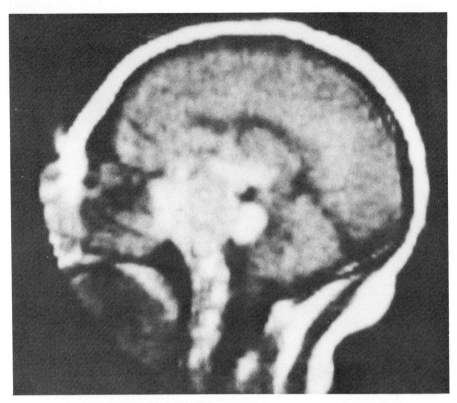

Figure 7-13. Chromophobe adenoma: SFFP. The full extent of the tumor upward, backward, and downward into the nasopharynx is easily appreciated in this sagittal image. (Reprinted with permission from Worthington, B.S.: Clinical prospects for nuclear magnetic resonance. Clin. Radiol. 34:3-12, 1983.)

Vascular Malformations

Tissue adjacent to an arteriovenous malformation may have abnormal T_1 and T_2 values and yield a different image intensity than normal parenchyma. Large vessels in the malformation may have rapid blood flow and appear dark. Small vessels frequently have slower flow and do not show significant flow effects. Vessels feeding the malformation and the rate of blood flow may be estimated. The Sturge-Webber syndrome has characteristic serpiginous vessels and associated parenchymal changes (8). MR has not been shown superior to contrast-enhanced CT in diagnosing arteriovenous malformations.

White Matter Diseases

MR is the first imaging modality capable of showing the normal myelination of white matter following birth (**Figure 7-14**). The optic radiations are myelinated during the first few months of life, followed by the principal sensory and motor tracts, the cerebral commissures, and the intracortical association areas (7). Once the range of normal

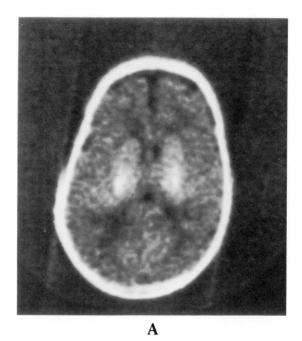

A

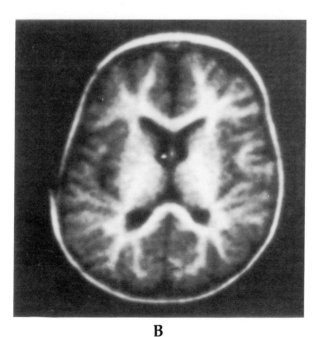

B

Figure 7-14. Normal myelination: IR. A, in a month-old infant, myelination has occurred only deep in the brain in the region of the posterior limb of the internal capsule. **B**, more extensive myelination is present in a year-old infant. (Reprinted with permission from Bydder, G.M.: Nuclear magnetic resonance of the brain. Appl. Radiol. Jan./Feb. 27-33, 1983.)

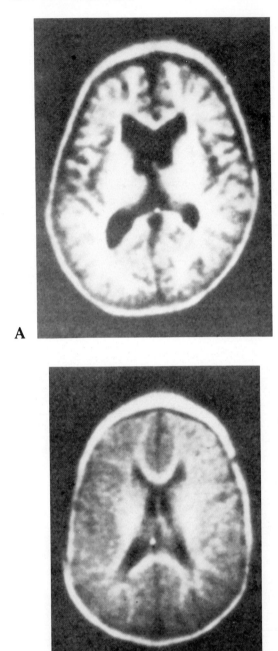

Figure 7-15. Mild hydrocephalus and probable rubella embryopathy: IR. A, the ventricular system is slightly dilated in an infant with hydrocephalus but the degree of myelination is normal. **B,** myelination appears to be delayed and asymmetric in the infant with rubella embryopathy. Both infants are 17 months old. (Reprinted with permission from Levene, M.E., and others: Nuclear magnetic imaging of the brain in children. Br. Med. J. 285:774-776, 1982.)

variation is determined, MR observations may be useful in the differential diagnosis and prognosis of developmental delays. Neonatal anoxic brain damage, rubella embryopathy, malnutrition, hypothyroidism, and phenylketonuria all affect myelination (22, 23) (**Figure 7-15**).

Autopsy studies of multiple sclerosis (MS) usually reveal many more lesions than were suspected on either clinical grounds or with CT. MR detects almost seven times as many lesions as does CT (20) (**Figure 7-16**). As many as 50% of patients with MS may have a normal

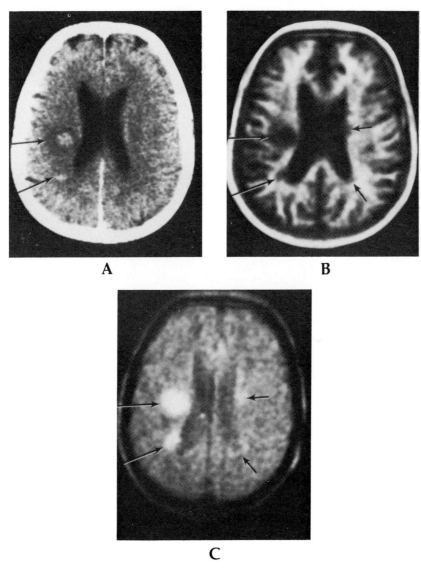

Figure 7-16. Multiple sclerosis. A, contrast-enhanced CT; **B**, IR; **C**, SE. Contrast-enhanced lesions in the CT scan are seen in both MR images (long arrows). Two other lesions were demonstrated only with MR (short arrows). (Reprinted with permission from Bydder, G.M., and others: Clinical NMR imaging of the brain: 140 cases. Am. J. Roentgenol. 139:215-236, 1982.)

CT and positive MR exam (4). Even when CT is positive, MR frequently shows more lesions. MR readily demonstrates lesions that are clinically silent, particularly in the brain stem (24).

Spin echo may be the most sensitive pulse sequence for detecting MS lesions (25). Multiple sclerosis can produce regions of prolonged T_1 and T_2 anywhere in the brain, although lesions are frequently periventricular. Lesions have high intensity in images obtained with a long TR/moderate TE SE sequence. In these images, lesions stand out clearly and false positives from partial volume effects are reduced. However, normal individuals sometimes have small regions of increased T_2 that can simulate MS plaques at the anterolateral angles of the lateral ventricles (**Figure 7-17**). False positives may be avoided by excluding lesions less than 3 x 3 mm and those with poorly defined margins (26). A cluster of small lesions may be difficult to distinguish from a single large lesion; this difficulty may be less of a problem with IR than with other pulse sequences.

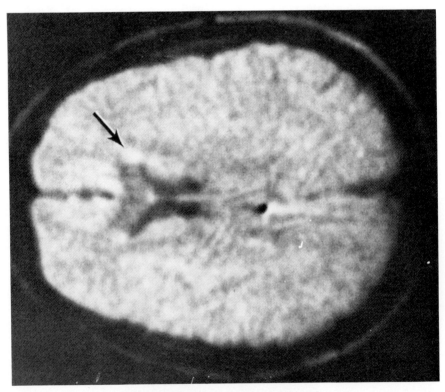

Figure 7-17. Normal brain: SE. A small region of increased T_2 is noted at the anterolateral angle of the lateral ventricle (arrow) and could be confused with a multiple sclerosis plaque unless strict criteria are used for differentiation. (Reprinted with permission from Young, I.R., Randell, C.P., and Kaplan, P.W.: Nuclear magnetic resonance [NMR] imaging in white matter disease of the brain using spin-echo sequences. J. Comput. Assist. Tomog. 7:290-294, 1983.)

Infection

MR is more sensitive than CT to inflammation and may permit diagnosis of the earliest stages of viral encephalitis (**Figure 7-18**) and abscess formation. CT is the imaging modality of choice for later stages of abscess because the capsule becomes visible following enhancement with iodinated contrast. Shrinkage of the capsule indicates a favorable response to antibiotics. MR usually cannot differentiate between the capsule and surrounding edema. However, the necrotic center of the abscess can be determined with MR (27) but not with CT. A necrotic center is important to identify if aspiration is being considered. More experience with MR will be necessary before it replaces CT in the evaluation of brain abscesses (27).

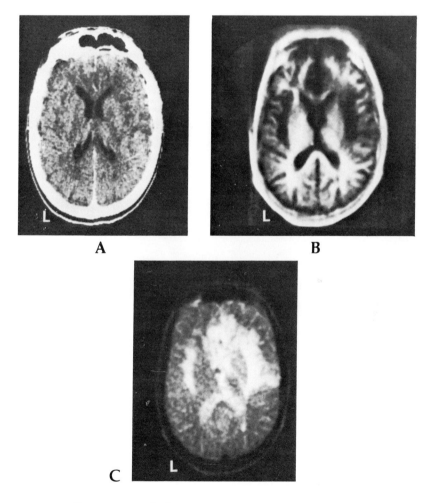

Figure 7-18. Herpes encephalitis. A, CT; **B**, IR; **C**, SE. Although all images reveal edema of the medial temporal lobes, it is easier to see with MR. The extent of disease is revealed best in the SE image. (Reprinted with permission from Bailes, D.R., and others: NMR imaging of the brain using spin-echo sequences. Clin. Radiol. 33:395-414, 1982.)

Posterior Fossa

The posterior fossa is surrounded by thick bone that limits access for biopsy and surgery and also limits the usefulness of CT. Improved accuracy is important in the diagnosis of posterior fossa diseases because a significant proportion of patients are treated on the basis of clinical and radiological findings alone (28). The posterior fossa can be examined by MR on essentially the same basis as the rest of the brain; the limitations of MR imaging in the posterior fossa are no different from those in the rest of the body. Bone destruction, bone erosion or sclerosis, and soft tissue calcification often are demonstrated better with CT than with MR. Contrast-enhanced CT is better for differentiating between tumor and surrounding edema (28).

The main advantages of MR over CT in the posterior fossa are increased sensitivity and more exact anatomical localization. In one small clinical series, almost 10% of tumors were not seen with CT but were detected with MR (28) (**Figure 7-19**). However, the overall sensitivity of MR to tumors in the posterior fossa is still unknown. In the majority of cases, the extent of posterior fossa tumors is depicted accurately by analysis of mass effects and the use of multiplanar imaging. Intrinsic tumors can usually be differentiated from extrinsic tumors more readily with MR than with CT (6, 28). The MR characteristics of fat make lipid components of tumors easier to identify (**Figure 7-20**); this property can provide diagnostic information in some cases.

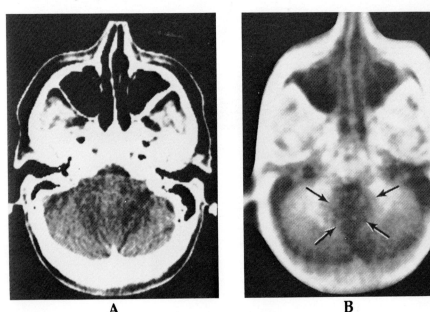

A   B

Figure 7-19. Intrinsic cerebellar tumor. A, contrast-enhanced CT; **B,** IR. The CT is normal, but the tumor is demonstrated in the IR image (arrows). (Reprinted with permission from Randell, C.P., and others: Nuclear magnetic resonance imaging of posterior fossa tumors. Am. J. Roentgenol. 141:489-496, 1983.)

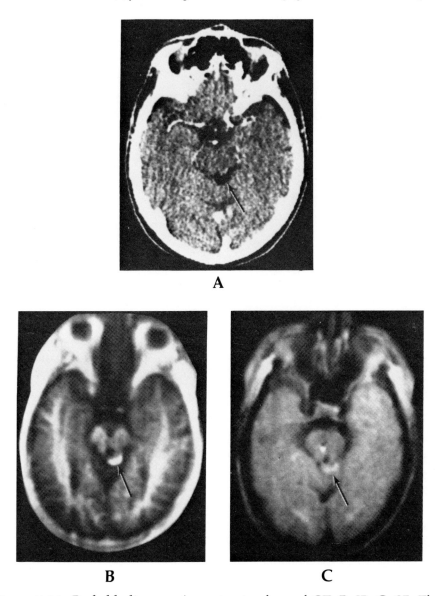

Figure 7-20. Probable lipoma. A, contrast-enhanced CT; **B,** IR; **C,** SE. The tumor is visible in all three images (arrows). It has increased intensity in the IR image because of a short T_1, and in the SE image because of an increased T_2. The high-intensity characteristics of MR make smaller lipid components more visible with MR compared to CT. (Reprinted with permission from Randell, C.P., and others: Nuclear magnetic resonance imaging of posterior fossa tumors. Am. J. Roentgenol. 141:489-496, 1983.)

The detection rate for brain stem and cerebellar infarctions is about 70 to 80% with MR (2), whereas most patients with brain stem infarcts have a normal CT (**Figure 7-21**). Inversion recovery images may be more sensitive than spin-echo for detection of small lesions (6). The detection rate of MR is also high for posterior fossa lesions caused by

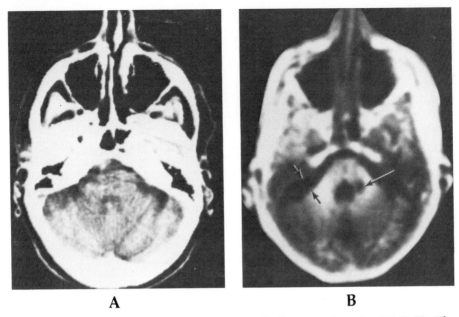

A   **B**

Figure 7-21. Brain stem infarction and cerebellar atrophy. A, CT; **B**, IR. The area of infarction appears dark (long arrow), and there is probable cerebellar atrophy (short arrows). The CT is normal. (Reprinted with permission from Bydder, G.M., and others: Clinical NMR imaging of the brain: 140 cases. Am. J. Roentgenol. 139:215-236, 1982.)

multiple sclerosis. MR may detect posterior fossa involvement in approximately 70 to 80% of MS patients; most of these patients yield a normal CT image (6, 24) (**Figure 7-22**). The shape of MS lesions often is irregular, with smaller lesions being circular or bar-shaped and larger ones following the direction of fiber tracts in the brain stem and middle cerebellar peduncles (24). In some patients with a suspected brain tumor, the detection of multiple lesions has led to the correct diagnosis of multiple sclerosis, with significant changes in prognosis and treatment.

The lack of signal from bone is helpful in the diagnosis of acoustic neuromas arising near or within the internal auditory canal and petrous bone. The increased T_1 of these tumors makes them hard to separate from the surrounding CSF and bone with inversion recovery imaging; however in SE images (**Figure 7-23**) they are highlighted against a dark background. Tumors of 8 mm have been detected (6), and smaller tumors potentially are detectable. Larger tumors are usually visible, and displacement of the pons and cerebellum are well demonstrated. The multiplanar capabilities of MR permit accurate size measurements of tumors prior to surgery; however, partial volume effects must be considered in these measurements (6).

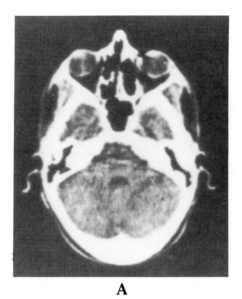

A

B

Figure 7-22. Multiple sclerosis. A, CT; **B**, IR. The CT image is normal, but four lesions (arrows) are seen within the pons and middle cerebellar peduncles in the IR image. The two small areas slightly to the right of the midline within the pons measure 2 mm by 2 mm and do not meet minimum size criteria for multiple sclerosis plaques in this study. (Reprinted with permission from Young, I.R., and others: Nuclear magnetic resonance of the brain in multiple sclerosis. Lancet, November 14:1063-1066, 1981.)

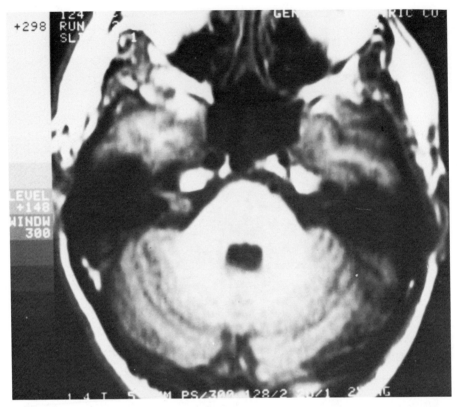

Figure 7-23. Acoustic neuroma: PS. The tumor in the right internal auditory canal stands out because it is surrounded by petrous bone with a low MR intensity. (Courtesy of General Electric Company.)

Spinal Cord

X-ray examination of the spinal cord requires intrathecal contrast. Clinical diagnosis of cervical cord lesions is difficult because conditions affecting the cervical cord may cause signs and symptoms that mimic the involvement of other parts of the central nervous system. In all likelihood, MR will become the imaging procedure of choice for examining the high cervical region because it clearly demonstrates the size, shape, and position of the cord without the use of a contrast agent.

Partial saturation images may provide the best spatial resolution and anatomic detail in the spinal cord (29). The sagittal plane is preferred for demonstrating the craniovertebral junction because it displays the brain stem, spinal cord, and fourth ventricle in the same image (30). The precise margin of the foramen magnum may be difficult to identify because cortical bone yields no MR signal. Its location must be inferred from the position of marrow in vertebral bodies, the odontoid process, and the clivus, and from soft tissue under the posterior margin (31). Although the depressed fourth ventricle and brain stem configuration of Chiari Type II malformations are shown clearly,

102

the exact position of the cerebellar tonsils relative to the foramen magnum frequently is not demonstrated (30). Despite these limitations, MR can be useful in assessing the position of the tip of the odontoid in basilar invagination, and the associated brain stem deformity is shown clearly (30) (**Figure 7-24**).

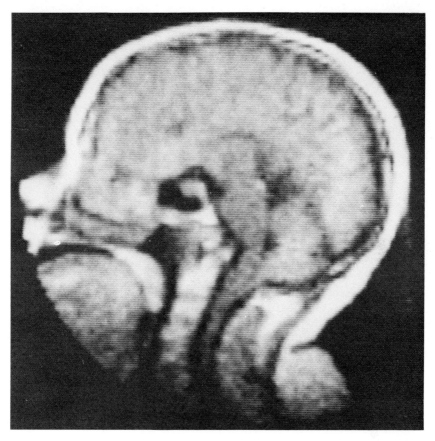

Figure 7-24. Basilar invagination: SSFP. The brain stem is deformed by the tip of an abnormally high odontoid process. (Reprinted with permission from Worthington, B.S.: Clinical prospects for nuclear magnetic resonance. Clin. Radiol. 34:3-12, 1983.)

Intrinsic tumors and syringomyelia both present with swelling of the spinal cord and can be difficult to differentiate even with metrizamide-enhanced CT studies (**Figure 7-25**). Since a syrinx contains fluid, it can be differentiated from a spinal cord tumor with MR (**Figure 7-26**). Sagittal images are superior in revealing the extent of the syrinx and in depicting the presence or absence of associated Arnold-Chiari malformations (30). Intrinsic tumors may have the same intensity as the spinal cord and may not be directly visible; however, the extent of the tumor often can be estimated from analysis of cord enlargement (29).

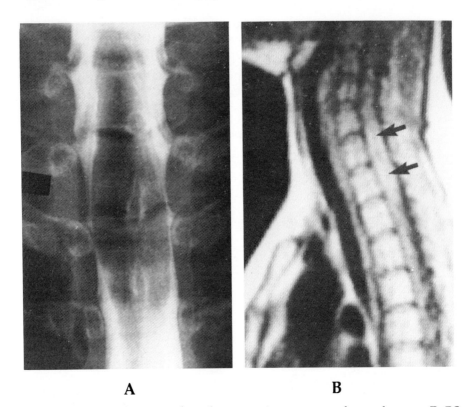

A   B

Figure 7-25. Intrinsic spinal cord tumor. A, metrizamide myelogram; **B**, PS. The myelogram shows fusiform enlargement of the spinal cord at the T_1-T_2 level. PS demonstrates the tumor mass and a central, cystic component (arrows). (Reprinted with permission from Han, J.S., and others: NMR imaging of the spine. Am. J. Neuroradiol. 4:1151-1159, 1983.)

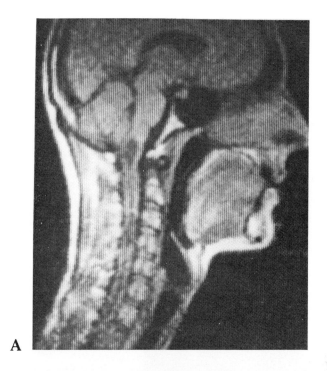

A

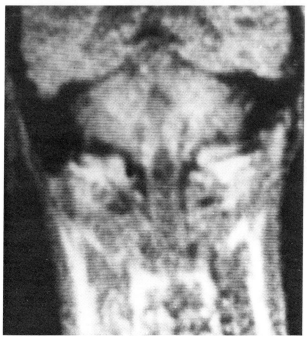

B

Figure 7-26. Cervicomedullary syrinx. A, sagittal and **B**, coronal SE. The syrinx is visible in both the sagittal and coronal images as an area of decreased signal intensity. The coronal image demonstrates communication of the fourth ventricle with the dilated cystic portion of the cervical cord. (Reprinted with permission from Modic, M.T., and others: Nuclear magnetic resonance imaging of the spine. Radiology 148:757-762, 1983.)

Lipomas have high intensity and stand out in most images. Sagittal sections are superior in demonstrating tethering of the cord (29) (**Figure 7-27**). Current equipment is not capable of differentiating gray and white matter in the spinal cord. Hence, MS lesions in the cord are very difficult to see (29).

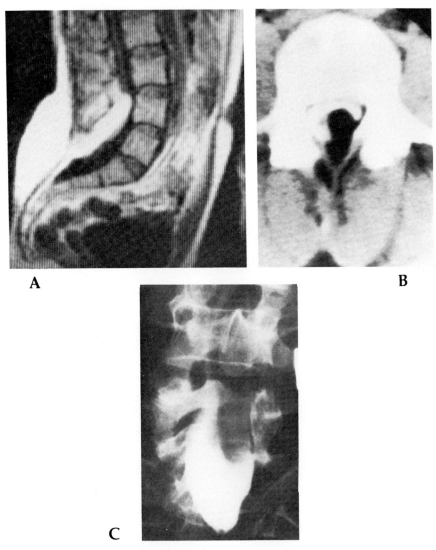

A   B

C

Figure 7-27. Lipoma and tethered cord. A, pantopaque myelogram. **B**, transverse high resolution CT with metrizamide. **C**, sagittal SE. The patient has a meningocele and urinary bladder dysfunction. The myelogram demonstrates a posterior defect in the contrast column. The CT shows a defect in the neural arch and an area of decreased attenuation impinging on the subarachnoid space posteriorly. The SE image shows cord tethering at the L3-4 level. The lipoma is high intensity and is continuous with the subcutaneous fat posterior to the neural arch defect. (Reprinted with permission from Modic, M.T., and others: Nuclear magnetic resonance imaging of the spine. Radiology 148:757-762, 1983.)

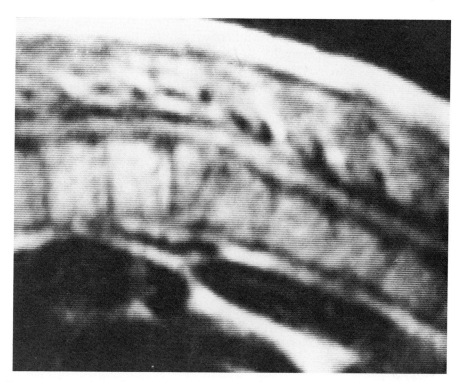

Figure 7-28. Spinal trauma: SE. The midthoracic vertebral segments are disrupted and impinge upon the spinal cord. The signal intensity and size of the cord are slightly increased superior to the lesion. The patient was paraplegic. (Reprinted with permission from Modic, M.T., and others: Nuclear magnetic resonance imaging of the spine. Radiology 148:757-762, 1983.)

In the spinal column, the vertebral bodies, discs, and spinal canal are well visualized. Discs have a central region of higher intensity surrounded by a region of lower intensity that is thought to represent the nucleus pulposus and annulus fibrosus. The cortex of vertebral bodies and the anterior and posterior longitudinal ligaments are all dark and cannot be distinguished. The lack of signal from cortical bone is a major drawback in the diagnosis of spinal stenosis and degenerative spurs, and causes MR to miss a significant number of abnormalities that are detectable by myelography (29). MR is inferior to CT in evaluation of the neural foramina and nerve roots because high spatial resolution and thin sections are not currently available with MR (31).

The ability to obtain images in different planes without moving the patient is extremely useful in cases of spinal cord trauma (31). However, MR is limited because bony and soft tissue fragments are difficult to see. Indirect evidence of spinal cord encroachment, such as abnormal cord size, shape, or position, sometimes provides diagnostic information. Swelling or disruption of the spinal cord usually is directly visible (**Figure 7-28**).

Spinal metastases may be visible with MR at a very early stage as a result of intensity changes in the marrow, and soft tissue extension can also be seen (29). MR may be as useful as contrast myelography in assessing spinal block (32). In addition, the location and extent of the block may be evaluated without injection of contrast in the cervical and lumbar regions (31).

References

1. Doyle, F.H., and others: Imaging of the brain by nuclear magnetic resonance. Lancet 11:53-57, 1981.
2. Bydder, G.M., and others: Clinical NMR imaging of the brain: 140 cases. Am. J. Roentgenol. 139:215-236, 1982.
3. Bydder, G.M.: Nuclear magnetic resonance of the brain. Appl. Radiol. Jan./Feb. 27-33, 1983.
4. Brant-Zawadzki, M., and others: NMR demonstration of cerebral abnormalities: Comparison with CT. Am. J. Roentgenol. 140:847-854, 1983.
5. Edelstein, W.A., and others: Signal, noise, and contrast in nuclear magnetic resonance (NMR) imaging. J. Comput. Assist. Tomog. 7:391-401, 1983.
6. Bydder, G.M., and others: Nuclear magnetic resonance imaging of the posterior fossa — 50 cases. Clin. Radiol. 34:173-188, 1983.
7. Simmonds, D., and others: NMR anatomy of the brain using inversion-recovery sequences. Neuroradiology 25:113-118, 1983.
8. Buonanno, F., and others: Clinical applications of nuclear magnetic resonance (NMR). Disease-a-Month 29:1-81, 1983.
9. Bryn, R.M., and others: Nuclear magnetic resonance evaluation of stroke. Radiology 149:189-192, 1983.
10. Crooks, L.E., and others: Clinical efficiency of nuclear magnetic resonance imaging. Radiology 146:123-128, 1983.
11. Spetzler, R.F., and others: Acute NMR changes during MCA occlusion; a preliminary study in primates. Stroke 14:185-191, 1983.
12. Levy, R.M., and others: NMR imaging of acute experimental cerebral ischemia: Time course and pharmacologic manipulations. Am. J. Neurol. Radiol. 4:238-241, 1983.
13. Mano, I., and others: Proton nuclear magnetic resonance imaging of acute experimental cerebral ischemia. Invest. Radiol. 18:345-351, 1983.
14. Hilal, S.K., and others: In vivo NMR imaging of tissue sodium in the intact cat before and after acute cerebral stroke. Am. J. Neurol. Radiol. 4:245-249, 1983.

15. Von Einsiedel, G.H., and Loffler, W.: Nuclear magnetic resonance imaging of brain tumors unrevealed by CT. Eur. J. Radiol. 2:225-234, 1982.

16. Steiner, R.E.: The Hammersmith clinical experience with nuclear magnetic resonance. Clin. Radiol. 34:13-23, 1983.

17. Brant-Zawadski, M., Mills, C.M., and Davis, P.L.: Applications of NMR to CNS disease. Appl. Radiol. Mar./Apr. 25-30, 1983.

18. Smith, F.W.: Whole body nuclear magnetic resonance imaging. Radiography 47:297-300, 1981.

19. Bailes, D.R., and others: NMR imaging of the brain using spin-echo sequences. Clin. Radiol. 33:395-414, 1982.

20. Margulis, A.R., and others: Nuclear magnetic resonance imaging clinical experience in San Francisco. Eur. J. Radiol. 3:236-238, 1983.

21. Hawkes, R.C., and others: The application of NMR imaging to the evaluation of pituitary and juxtasellar tumors. Am. J. Neurol. Radiol. 4:221-222, 1983.

22. Levene, M.I., and others: Nuclear magnetic imaging of the brain in children. Br. Med. J. 285:774-776, 1982.

23. Henderson, R.G.: Nuclear magnetic resonance imaging: a review. J. Roy. Soc. Med. 76:206-212, 1983.

24. Young, I.R., and others: Nuclear magnetic resonance of the brain in multiple sclerosis. Lancet 14:1063-1066, 1981.

25. Lukes, S.A., and others: Nuclear magnetic resonance imaging in multiple sclerosis. Ann. Neurol. 13:592-601, 1983.

26. Young, I.R., Randell, C.P., and Kaplan, P.W.: Nuclear magnetic resonance (NMR) imaging in white matter disease of the brain using spin-echo sequences. J. Comput. Assist. Tomog. 7:290-294, 1983.

27. Brant-Zawadski, M., and others: NMR imaging of experimental brain abscess: Comparison with CT. Am. J. Neurol. Radiol. 4:250-253, 1983.

28. Randell, C.P., and others: Nuclear magnetic resonance imaging of posterior fossa tumors. Am. J. Roentgenol. 141:489-496, 1983.

29. Han, J.S., and others: NMR imaging of the spine. Am. J. Neurol. Radiol. 4:1151-1159, 1983.

30. Hawkes, R.C., and others: Craniovertebral junction pathology: Assessment with NMR. Am. J. Neurol. Radiol. 4:232-233, 1983.

31. DeLaPaz, R.L., and others: Nuclear magnetic resonance (NMR) imaging of Arnold-Chiari Type I malformation with hydromyelia. J. Comput. Assist. Tomog. 7:126-129, 1983.

32. Modic, M.T., and others: Nuclear magnetic resonance imaging of the spine. Radiology 148:757-762, 1983.

33. Sipponen, J.T., and others: Nuclear magnetic resonance [NMR] imaging of intracerebral hemorrhage in the acute and resolving phases. J. Comput. Assist. Tomog. 7:954-959, 1983.

Chapter 8
Magnetic Resonance Imaging of the Body

Neck

Multiplanar MR imaging techniques are especially useful in the neck. Because of the superior soft tissue contrast of MR, individual muscles, cartilage, and blood vessels are revealed and the larynx and tongue base are shown well (**Figures 8-1** and **8-2**). Primary neck tumors, lymphomas, and angiofibromas are demonstrated clearly (1) without artifact from dental material (**Figures 8-3** and **8-4**). MR depicts many tissue abnormalities before size or shape distortions occur; often tumor infiltration and metastatic lymph nodes are shown more clearly with MR than with CT. Partial or complete obstruction of blood flow in the internal jugular vein occurs with some large neck tumors; MR can often detect these flow abnormalities (2) (**Figure 8-5**).

Mediastinum, Hila, and Lung Parenchyma

Solid tumors such as thyroid carcinoma can be differentiated from colloid cysts by differences in T_1 and T_2 (1). Measurements of T_1 have been useful in differentiating autonomous nodules, thyroiditis, and carcinoma; however, there is often some overlap in the T_1 values (7).

The entire extent of the aorta, the great arteries arising from the arch, the subclavian, brachiocephalic and azygos veins, and the vena cava are all visible with MR. Also demonstrable are the spine, spinal cord, and intercostal and chest wall muscles. The main pulmonary artery and its proximal branches and the pulmonary veins as they enter the left atrium are routinely visible (**Figure 8-6**). These structures can be distinguished from tumors, lymph nodes, and other hilar structures without contrast administration (**Figure 8-7**). Lymph nodes smaller than 1 cm, and calcified nodes that are obvious in CT images, are not routinely visible with MR (4). Central and peripheral parenchymal nodules greater than about 1 cm are easily detected with MR. Respiratory and cardiac motion may interfere with visualization of nodules at the lung bases; this potential problem has not been systematically evaluated (5).

In about 25% of patients examined in a small series (4), hilar and mediastinal disease was better characterized by MR than by contrast-

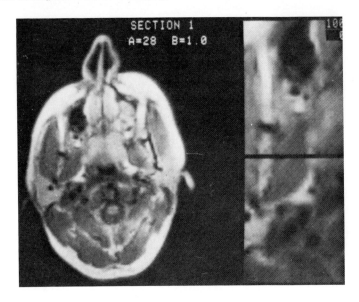

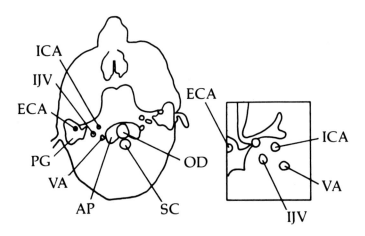

Figure 8-1. Upper neck: SE. The internal carotid artery (ICA), internal jugular vein (IJV), parotid gland (PG), external carotid artery (ECA), vertebral artery (VA), articulating process of C_1 (AP), spinal cord (SC), and odontoid process (OD) are all clearly shown. Also shown is inflammatory disease of the maxillary sinus (not labeled). (Reprinted with permission from Crooks, L., and others: Nuclear magnetic resonance whole body imager operating at 3.5 KGauss. Radiology 143:169-174, 1982.)

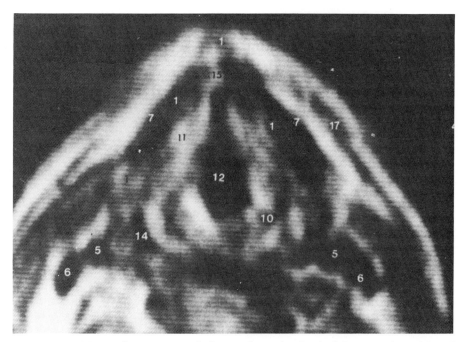

Figure 8-2. Normal anatomy of the neck at the high false vocal cord level: SE. Thyroid cartilage (1), common carotid artery (5), jugular vein (6), strap muscles (7), arytenoid cartilages (10), false vocal cords (11), laryngeal vestibule (12), pyriform sinus (14), pre-epiglottic space (15), and platysma muscle (17). (Reprinted with permission from Lufkin, R.B., and others: NMR anatomy of the larynx and tongue base. Radiology, 148:173-175, 1983.)

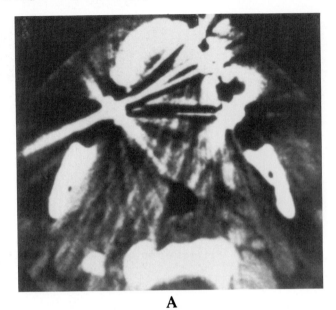

A

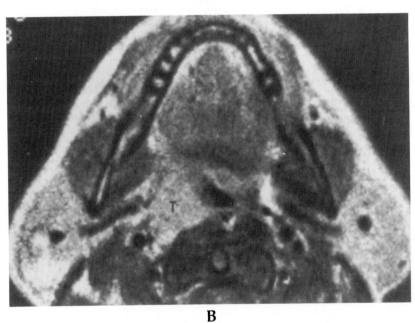

B

Figure 8-3. Nasopharyngeal carcinoma. A, CT; **B,** SE. Artifact from dental fillings obscure the tumor with CT. With MR the tumor (T) is seen to extend to the right glossopharyngeal sulcus. (Reprinted with permission from Dillon W.P., and deGroot, J.: Nasopharynx. In Margulis, A.R., and others, editors: Clinical Magnetic Resonance Imaging. San Francisco: 1983, Radiology Research and Education Foundation.)

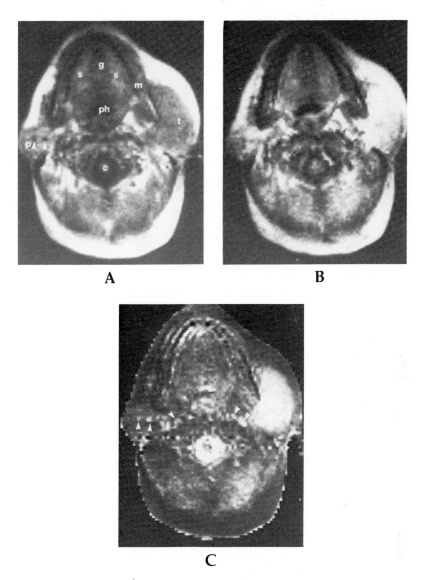

Figure 8-4. Parotid gland sarcoma: SE and calculated T₁ images. A, the tumor (t) has moderate to low intensity in the short TR/moderate TE spin-echo sequence. Normal anatomy is well demonstrated: g = genioglossus muscle, s = sublingual gland, m = mandible, ph = pharynx, p = parotid gland, c = spinal cord, arrowheads = external and internal carotid arteries and jugular veins. Behind the mandible the tumor is infiltrating medially toward the pterygopalatine groove. **B,** the tumor is imaged with increased intensity in the long TR/moderate TE image. **C,** increased intensity in the T₁ image indicates the prolonged T₁ of the tumor. (Reprinted with permission from Rupp, N., Reiser, M., and Stetter, E.: The diagnostic value of morphology and relaxation times in NMR imaging of the body. Eur. J. Radiol. 3:68-76, 1983.)

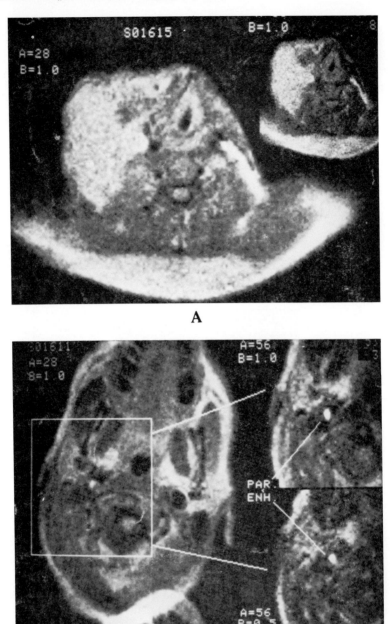

A

B

Figure 8-5. Large squamous cell carcinoma of the right neck: SE. A, the tumor displaces the right jugular vein and right internal carotid artery. **B,** shows increased intensity of the right jugular vein because of decreased blood flow from obstruction by the tumor. The intensity of the jugular vein is increased on the second echo. This effect has been called "paradoxical enhancement" (PAR ENH). (Reprinted with permission from Crooks, L.E., Mills, C.M., and Davis, P.L.: Visualization of cerebral and vascular abnormalities by NMR imaging: Effects of imaging parameters on contrast. Radiology 144:843-852, 1982.)

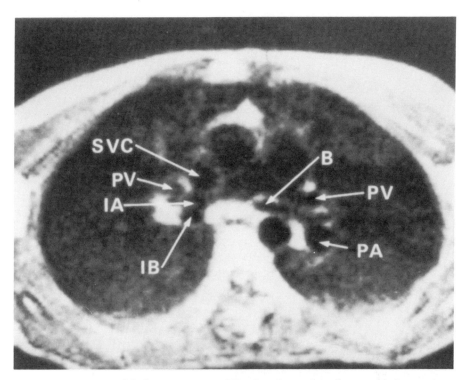

Figure 8-6. Normal hilar anatomy: SE. On the right, the interlobar pulmonary artery (IA) is anterior to the intermediate bronchus (IB) and behind the superior vena cava (SVC). The superior pulmonary vein (PV) is lateral. On the left, the main bronchus (B) is visible behind the pulmonary vein (PV) and anterior to the descending pulmonary artery (PA). The intense signal in both hila is from hilar fat. (Reprinted with permission from Gamsu, G., and others: Nuclear magnetic resonance imaging of the thorax. Radiology 147:473-480, 1983.)

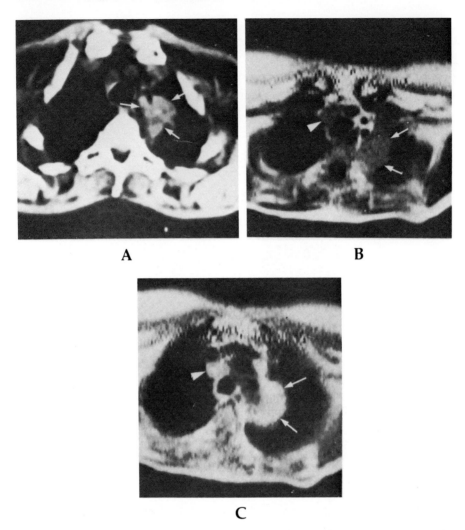

Figure 8-7. Bronchogenic carcinoma. A, CT; **B** and **C**, SE. The tumor mass is visible with CT (arrows). The MR images show the mass and a mediastinal lymph node (arrowheads). This metastatic node was thought to be a vessel in the CT image. The intensity in both short TR (**B**) and moderate TR (**C**) images, and the intensity increase in the moderate TR image, indicate the true nature of the structure. (Reprinted with permission from Cohen, A.M., and others: NMR evaluation of hilar and mediastinal lymphadenopathy. Radiology 148:739-742, 1983.)

enhanced CT. Tumor deposits and metastatic nodes often can be distinguished from hilar blood vessels in magnetic resonance images, and the extent of primary tumors and invasion of vessels are shown more clearly. Sometimes it is difficult to distinguish tumor mass or lymphadenopathy from mediastinal fat; in these cases inversion recovery or short TR spin-echo images may be helpful (4). Unfortunately, T_1 and T_2 values do not reliably permit differentiation of benign from malignant tumors, benign from malignant adenopathy, or pneumonia, atelectasis, and empyema one from the other (3). It may be possible to distinguish transudates, exudates, and empyema on the basis of T_1 measurements, because the T_1 value appears to be related to protein content (1).

Cardiovascular Studies

Cardiac motion does not produce artifacts in ungated studies but may cause a loss of spatial resolution in the image. The greatest loss of detail occurs in normal young patients who exhibit the greatest amplitude of ventricular contraction. The ventricular walls and interatrial and interventricular septa can sometimes be seen in ungated images. The vena cava, aorta, pulmonary arteries, and pulmonary veins are usually visible.

EKG activity can be used to trigger data acquisition in MR (gating), and images can be formed over many cardiac cycles from data accumulated during selected 50-msec portions of each cycle. Gated images improve spatial resolution significantly at the expense of some increase in imaging time. Valves and valve leaflets, papillary muscles, chordae tendinae (**Figure 8-8**), the moderator band, and the endocardium, myocardium, and pericardium (**Figure 8-9**) are shown clearly, and moving blood provides excellent contrast. Filling defects such as mural thrombus and valve vegetations can be seen. Gating also permits measurement of myocardial T_1 and T_2, myocardial thickness, and the dimensions of the chambers at systole and diastole. From the latter measurements, the stroke volume and the ejection fraction can be calculated. Proximal portions of the coronary arteries and coronary artery grafts can sometimes be visualized (5) (**Figure 8-10**); visualization of these structures should improve if surface coils are developed specifically for cardiac imaging. Eventually, MR combined with blood flow measurements may prove useful in assessing atherosclerotic coronary artery disease and graft patency.

Gated images can be used to evaluate congenital heart disease (6) (**Figures 8-11** and **8-12**). Ventricular hypertrophy, atretic and stenotic valves, poststenotic dilatation, and transposition of the great vessels have been observed with MR. Ventricular septal defects are usually apparent, but atrial septal defects may be hard to distinguish from the normally thin interatrial septum, and small defects may not be detectable.

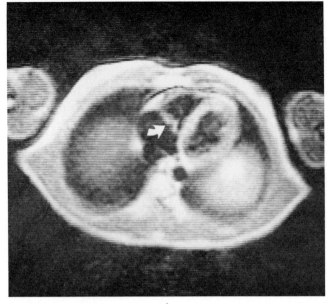

A

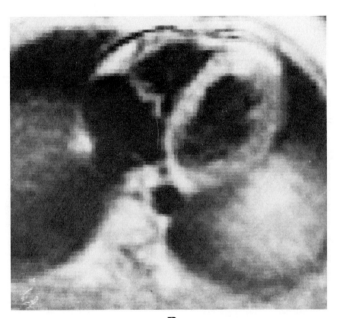

B

Figure 8-8. Normal cardiac anatomy: gated SE. A, the tricuspid valve (arrow), right atrium, right ventricle, left ventricle, the papillary muscles, and the aorta are seen. **B**, the expanded view shows these structures in greater detail. (Reprinted with permission from Alfidi, R.J., and others: Preliminary results in humans and animals with a superconducting whole body nuclear magnetic resonance. Radiology 143:175-181, 1982.)

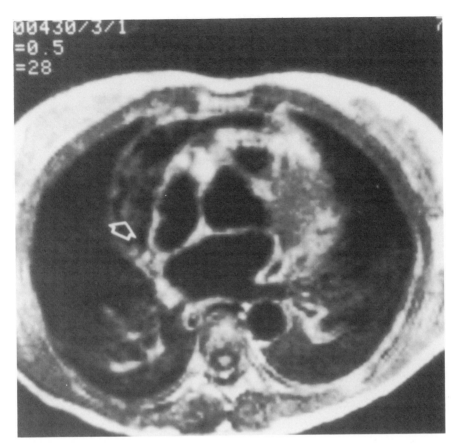

Figure 8-9. Uremic pericarditis: gated SE. An asymmetric and presumably loculated effusion is evident over the right side of the heart. The regions of higher intensity within this effusion (open arrow) may arise from inflammatory debris within the effusion. (Reprinted with permission from Higgins, C.B., and others: Nuclear magnetic resonance imaging of the cardiovascular system. Radiographics 4:122-136, 1984.)

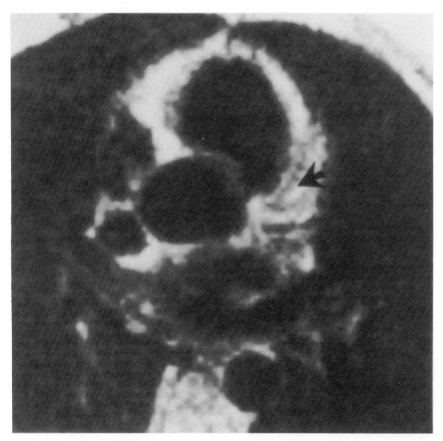

Figure 8-10. Normal coronary artery: gated SE. The proximal portion of the left anterior descending coronary artery (arrow) is demonstrated. (Reprinted with permission from Higgins, C.B., and others: Nuclear magnetic resonance imaging of the cardiovascular system. Radiographics 4:122-136, 1984.)

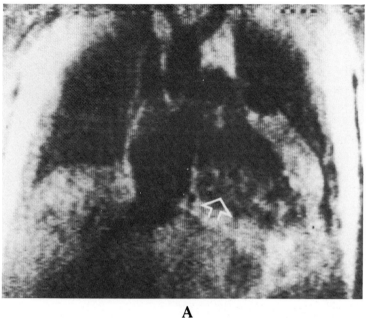

A

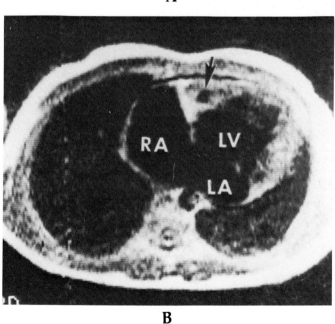

B

Figure 8-11. Tricuspid atresia: gated SE. A, the coronal section demonstrates the heavily trabeculated, thickened wall of the hypoplastic right ventricle (arrow). The right atrium is enlarged. Normal anatomical relationships of the superior vena cava, ascending aorta, pulmonary artery, and left atrial appendage are also shown. **B,** in the transverse section the atrial septum is almost entirely absent. The area of the atretic tricuspid valve is thickened, and the right ventricular cavity is hypoplastic (arrow). The mitral valve, right atrium (RA), left atrium (LA), and left ventricle (LV) are normal. (Reprinted with permission from Fletcher, B.D., and others: Gated magnetic resonance imaging of congenital cardiac malformation. Radiology 150:137-140, 1984.)

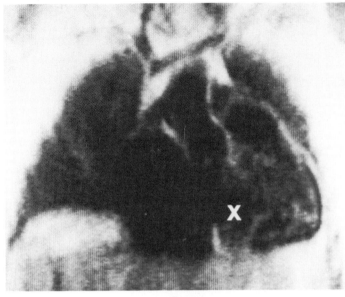

A

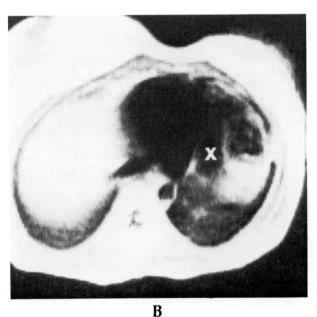

B

Figure 8-12. Ebstein's anomaly: gated SE: The "atrialized" portion of the
right ventricle (X) can be seen between a dilated tricuspid valve and abnormal
valve leaflets in both the coronal, **A**, and axial, **B**, sections. Normal aortic valve
leaflets are visible in **A**. (Reprinted with permission from Fletcher, B.D., and
others: Gated magnetic resonance imaging of congenital cardiac malformation. Radiology 150:137-140, 1984.)

Three-dimensional (3-D) data acquisition facilitates the display of cardiac anatomy because any desired imaging plane can be selected; however each 3-D scan may take an hour (6). Eventually MR may contribute in a significant way to the evaluation of congenital heart disease, especially if the spatial resolution of magnetic resonance images can be improved.

MR evaluation of myocardial infarction is promising. Within 90 minutes of coronary artery ligation, changes in the myocardium consistent with intracellular edema can be detected by light microscopy (7). Immediate and delayed increases in T_1 and T_2 related to edema have been found in infarcted muscle (8, 9) and myocardial infarctions have been seen in T_2 weighted images (10) (**Figure 8-13**). Several indirect signs have also been observed. Ischemic myocardium moves more slowly and produces a stronger signal in ungated images. Blood flow adjacent to the damaged myocardium may be sluggish or turbulent and yield a stronger MR signal (7); also, adherent intraluminal blood clots may be seen in gated images (**Figure 8-14**). Spectroscopy, spectroscopic imaging, and new contrast agents may lead to even greater sensitivity and specificity in the detection and evaluation of the severity of myocardial infarction.

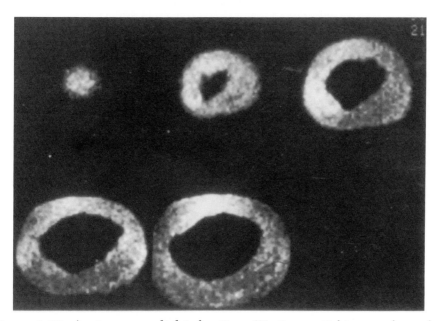

Figure 8-13. Acute myocardial infarction: SE. Sequential images from the apex to the midportion in the left ventricle of a dog demonstrate increased myocardial intensity due to T_2 prolongation. These images were obtained 24 hours after ligation of the left anterior descending artery. (Reprinted with permission from Higgins, C.B., and others: Cardiovascular system. In Margulis, A.R., and others, editors: Clinical Magnetic Resonance Imaging. San Francisco: 1983, Radiology Research and Education Foundation.)

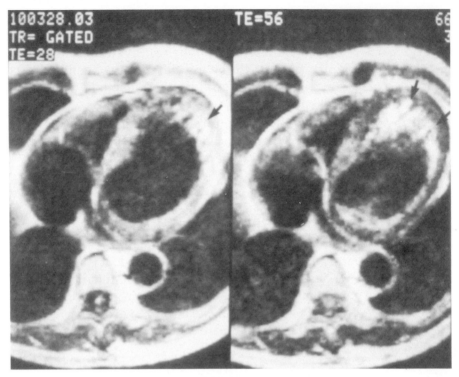

Figure 8-14. Old anterior myocardial infarction: gated SE. A mural thrombosis (arrows) is demonstrated in the anterior portion of the left ventricle. The thrombus produces high-signal intensity and can be distinguished from the myocardium. Discrimination of thrombus from myocardium is provided better in the second echo image (moderate TE). Some of the high intensity adjacent to the anterior wall may be due to sluggish flow as well as to the thrombus. (Reprinted with permission from Higgins, C.B., and others: Nuclear magnetic resonance imaging of the cardiovascular system. Radiographics 4:122-136, 1984.)

MR can differentiate between the lipid and connective tissue components of atherosclerotic carotid and femoral arteries and reveal the extent of lumenal narrowing (11, 12) (**Figure 8-15**); however, a systematic study of these arteries has not yet been performed. The extent of aortic atherosclerotic disease can be assessed by MR and lesion components can be differentiated; however, calcification is not always visible (12) (**Figure 8-16**). Aortic aneurysms and dissections can be evaluated without contrast media. The true and false lumens, intimal flaps, and thrombus may be seen clearly (**Figure 8-17**), and multiplanar imaging helps demonstrate whether the dissection extends to the renal arteries.

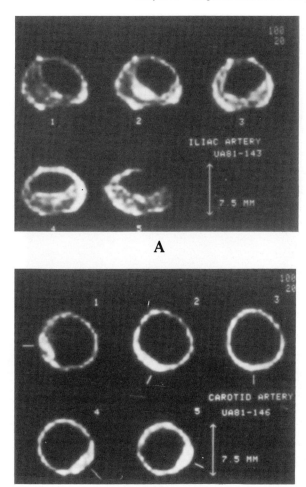

Figure 8-15. Atherosclerotic plaques: images of contiguous sections of excised arteries. A, in the iliac lesion two separate components are visible. Dense connective tissue appears dark (sections 1, 4, and 5) and surrounds a lipid portion, which appears white (sections 2 and 3). The mixture of connective tissue and lipid portions signifies advanced disease. **B,** the carotid lesions contain a more homogeneous blend of lipid and connective tissue. (Reprinted with permission from Kaufman, L., and others: The potential impact of nuclear magnetic resonance imaging on cardiovascular diagnosis. Circulation 67:251-257, 1983.)

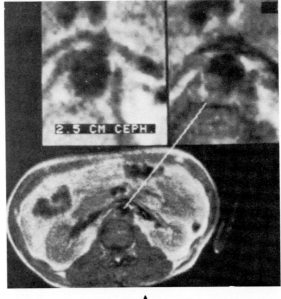

A

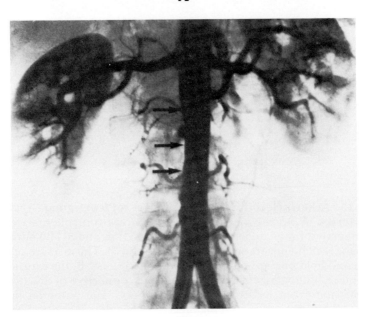

B

Figure 8-16. Aortic atherosclerosis. A, arteriogram. B, SE. The SE images reveal an atherosclerotic plaque projecting into the aortic lumen. Insets contain magnified views of the aorta at the level of the lesion and at a level 2.5 cm cephalad. The aortagram confirms the atherosclerotic narrowing of the aorta (arrows). (Reprinted with permission from Herfkens, R.J., and others: Nuclear magnetic resonance imaging of atherosclerotic disease. Radiology 148:161-166, 1983.)

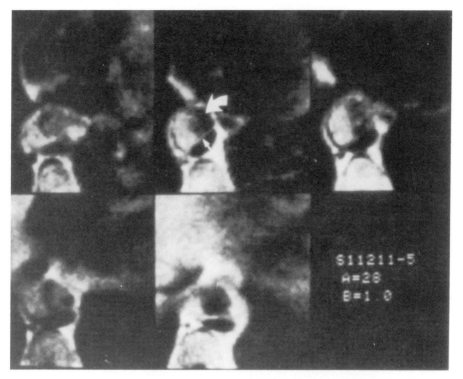

A

Figure 8-17. Type B aortic dissection. A, MR image; **B,** angiography. Spin-echo images through the lower descending aorta show a thrombus in the false channel (curved arrows), and no signal in the true lumen because of flowing blood. The intimal flap is also visible (arrow). Equally diagnostic information is available from the angiogram but at increased risk to the patient from catheterization and injection of contrast material. (Reprinted with permission from Herfkens, R.J., and others: Nuclear magnetic resonance imaging of the cardiovascular system; normal and pathologic findings. Radiology 147:749-759, 1983.)

see **B** on next page

129

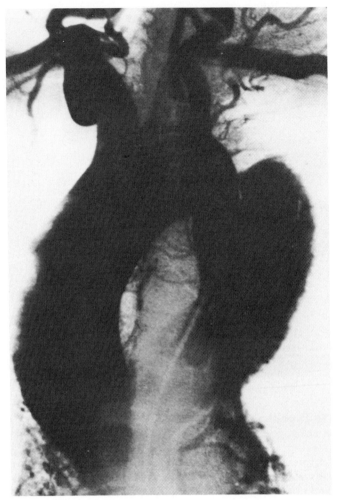

Figure 8-17.   **B**

Breast

In breast imaging with MR, the patient usually is imaged prone with the breasts freely suspended between foam supports to minimize the effects of respiratory motion and to spread the tissues. Compared to x-ray mammography, MR has the advantages of planar imaging and superior soft tissue resolution. It also does not require exposure to ionizing radiation. Fat and other soft tissues are readily differentiated, and cysts have a characteristic appearance. Dysplastic breasts are variable in appearance, with T_1 values that encompass a wide range and overlap the values characteristic of carcinoma (13, 14). Age, number of pregnancies, history of breast feeding, use of exogenous hormones, and the menstrual cycle may all affect T_1. More experience is needed before the sensitivity and specificity of MR in the detection of breast cancer is known. MR may be useful in tumor staging since infiltration of the tumor into the chest wall and axilla has been visualized (15).

Abdomen

The spatial resolution of abdominal MR images is comparable to those obtained with CT, although there is some resolution loss from respiratory movement near the diaphragm. The superior soft tissue contrast of MR compensates in part for poorer spatial resolution and increases the detectability of small lesions. The tissue yielding the most intense MR signal is fat, followed by viscera, muscle, fluid-filled cavities, bone, and air. Lung parenchyma is dark because of its air content. Usually the small bowel and colon have a uniform gray appearance; however, they may be dark if they contain air or fluid. Surrounding fat helps to delineate most organs and vessels (**Figures 8-18** and **8-19**). Because of its longer T_1, the spleen is darker than the liver in inversion recovery or T_1-weighted spin-echo images, and the vascular pedicle of the spleen usually can be seen entering the hilum (16). The spinal cord can be identified within the spinal canal, surrounded by CSF. Individual muscles such as the psoas and paraspinal can be readily identified.

A number of blood vessels are visible because of the contrast provided by flowing blood. These vessels serve as anatomical markers for identifying normal organs and mass effects. The inferior vena cava is so well demonstrated that changes in its shape and caliber are easily appreciated at the level of the renal veins and within the liver (17). MR may be superior to all other imaging modalities, including angiography, in demonstrating dilatation of the splenic vein in portal hypertension (16) (**Figure 8-20**). It is often superior to ultrasound in revealing vascular structures because it is free of interference from bowel gas. Multiplanar imaging is particularly useful for demonstrating the aorta and vena cava and their major tributaries. Future applications may include the evaluation of cirrhosis, portocaval shunts, vascular invasion by tumors, and renal vascular malformations (17).

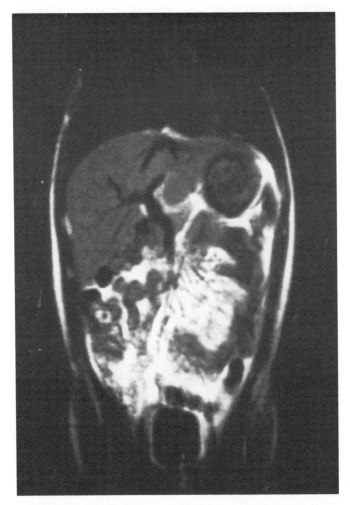

Figure 8-18. Normal abdominal anatomy: coronal PS. Branches of the superior mesenteric artery are visible as dark, linear structures in white mesenteric fat in the left mid-abdomen. The superior mesenteric vein extends vertically and is continuous with the portal vein and its intrahepatic branches. The confluence of hepatic veins is visible just below the diaphragm near the midline. The fundus of the stomach is the round structure just below the left hemidiaphragm. Moderate intensity linear structures surrounded by fat are small bowel loops and portions of the colon. Bowel gas is black. The midline structure at the bottom of the image is the bladder; this structure is dark because of the long T_1 of urine. (Courtesy of General Electric Company.)

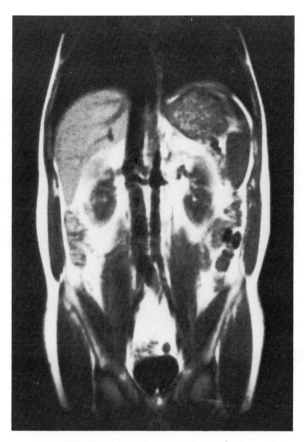

Figure 8-19. Normal abdominal anatomy: coronal PS. The full length of the vena cava, most of the abdominal aorta, and proximal portions of the renal arteries are dmonstrated in this image. The kidneys are outlined by fat, and the renal cortex and medulla can be distinguished. The darker structure just below and lateral to the stomach is a portion of the spleen. Muscles are imaged with moderately low intensity. The psoas muscles are seen running vertically on either side of the midline in the lower half of the image. (Courtesy of General Electric Company.)

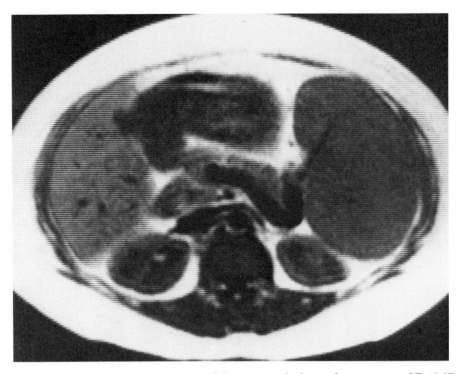

Figure 8-20. Splenomegaly and dilatation of the splenic vein: SR. MR appears to delineate the vascular system better than any other modality. (Reprinted with permission from Borkowski, G.P., and others: Nuclear magnetic resonance [NMR] imaging in the evaluation of the liver; preliminary experience. J. Comput. Assist. Tomog. 7:768-784, 1983.)

The superior soft tissue discrimination of MR is helpful in evaluating abdominal masses. Cysts are readily distinguished from solid tumors by MR, even when the CT examination is equivocal. Definition of the extent of lesions is often facilitated by sagittal or coronal images. As with head and neck tumors, infiltration and metastatic nodes should be easier to see, and MR may become the modality of choice for preoperative staging of some tumors, particularly those in the pelvis.

In some patients, streak artifacts from surgical clips and air-fluid levels in the stomach or bowel obscure lesions in the CT images (**Figure 8-21**). The absence of clip artifacts in magnetic resonance images may be an advantage in monitoring for tumor recurrence following surgery. Lesions in the liver periphery may be easier to see with MR because of the absence of artifacts from adjacent ribs (**Figure 8-22**). The difficulty in seeing calcifications in MR is a disadvantage in some cases.

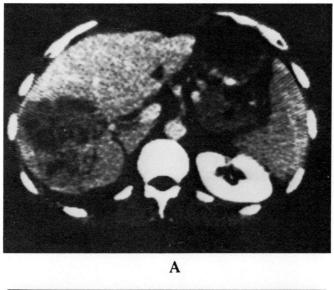

A

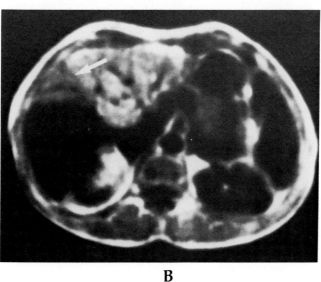

B

Figure 8-21. Hepatoma. A, contrast-enhanced CT; B, IR. The hepatoma is clearly visible in both images, although the inversion recovery image offers greater contrast. The IR image also shows a wedge-shaped area of infarction (arrow) just anterior to the tumor; this area is not visible in the CT image. (Reprinted with permission from Doyle, F.H., and others: Nuclear magnetic resonance imaging of the liver; initial experience. Am. J. Roentgenol. 138:193-200, 1982.)

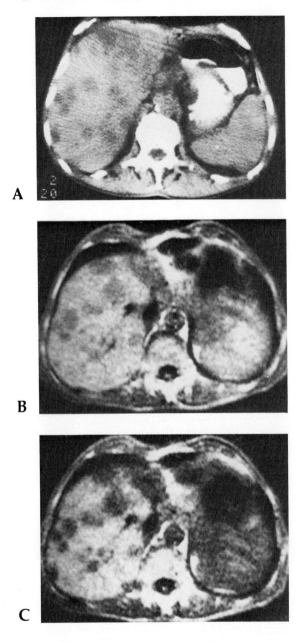

Figure 8-22. Metastatic colon carcinoma. A, CT; **B,** SE; **C,** IR. Multiple defects are present in the liver. The metastases have prolonged T_1 values and decreased intensity in the short TR/short TE spin-echo and inversion recovery images. A lesion visible in the posterior aspect of the right lobe of the liver could be confused with rib artifact in the CT image. (Reprinted with permission from Borkowski, G.P., and others: Nuclear magnetic resonance [NMR] imaging in the evaluation of the liver; preliminary experience. J. Comput. Assist. Tomog. 7:768-784, 1983.)

Liver

The hepatic veins are routinely seen within the liver at their confluence with the inferior vena cava (IVC), and the portal vein and its branches are readily visible as dark structures within the liver parenchyma. As in CT, nonobstructed intrahepatic biliary ducts are usually not visible. Obstructed ducts can be differentiated from portal veins by flow-dependent sequences, including partial saturation images. Frequently the level of obstruction can be demonstrated. Dilated venous collaterals in alcohol-related cirrhosis are easier to appreciate with MR than with CT (16).

MR depicts focal liver lesions with a sensitivity comparable to CT. Hepatomas are shown with greater contrast with MR, and the tumor margins are more clearly defined than with CT (**Figure 8-23**). MR is superior in demonstrating the internal structure of the hepatoma and its relationship to hepatic vessels (18), and may be the modality of choice for differentiating necrotic tumor from other cystic lesions (19). In a significant number of cases, however, it may not be possible to distinguish hepatomas from large metastatic lesions or benign conditions such as adenomas (18).

Inversion recovery images and long TR spin-echo images may provide the highest lesion contrast for liver imaging. Hepatomas have long T_1 and T_2 values, with greater variability in the T_1 values. Metastases may have a normal T_2, but the T_1 values are usually prolonged (15). Prolonged relaxation times are also found in hepatitis, abscesses, infarction, hematomas, and other conditions; therefore, the appearance of a lesion in a magnetic resonance image may not suggest a specific diagnosis. Determination of absolute T_1 and T_2 values may not increase diagnostic specificity because these parameters may not discriminate primary from metastatic tumors or tumors from benign conditions.

MR may reveal diffuse parenchymal disease earlier than CT or ultrasound in some cases because biochemical changes frequently precede alterations in liver morphology. Clinical data are insufficient to evaluate this possibility. Fatty infiltration does not consistently alter T_1 and T_2 values; although the liver may have a slightly altered intensity in MR, CT numbers are more dependable than T_1 measurements in revealing fatty infiltration (20). In some cases of primary biliary cirrhosis and hemochromatosis, the deposition of paramagnetic copper and iron shortens both T_1 and T_2. Although MR has been reported to be both sensitive and specific in revealing low levels of iron (18), the liver may still look normal in hemochromatosis because fibrosis prolongs T_1 (16). Alcoholic cirrhosis (**Figure 8-24**) and viral hepatitis are frequently detectable because of a significantly prolonged T_1 (20) that distinguishes these conditions from fatty infiltration.

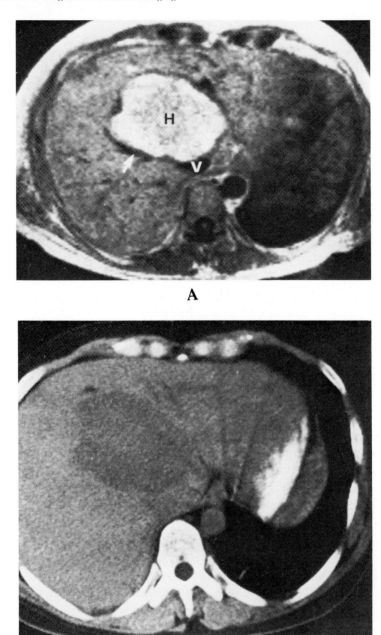

A

B

Figure 8-23. Hepatoma. A, SE; B, CT. The hepatoma has high intensity in the SE image. Its internal structure and surrounding capsule are well delineated and it displaces but does not obstruct the inferior vena cava (V) and portal vein (arrow). The hepatoma's internal architecture, capsule, and relationship to hepatic vascular structures are poorly delineated in the CT image. (Reprinted with permission from Moss, A.A., and others: Liver, gallbladder, alimentary tube, spleen, peritoneal cavity, and pancreas. In Margulis, A.R., and others, editors: Clinical Magnetic Resonance Imaging. San Francisco: 1983, Radiology Research and Education Foundation.)

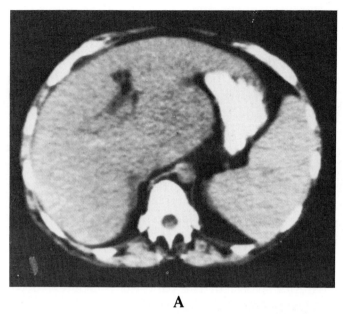

A

B

Figure 8-24. Alcoholic cirrhosis. A, CT; B, IR. The CT scan is normal. The MR image shows the liver to be diffusely abnormal and dark because of prolonged T_1. (Reprinted with permission from Doyle, F.H., and others: Nuclear magnetic resonance imaging of the liver; initial experience. Am. J. Roentgenol. 138:193-200, 1982.)

Bile in the intrahepatic ducts produces a low-intensity spin-echo signal; when it is concentrated by the gallbladder, however, it yields a higher intensity signal because T_1 becomes relatively short. Following the stimulation of normal individuals with a fatty meal, low-intensity bile may be seen floating on a layer of residual bile of higher MR intensity. MR may be the first modality capable of evaluating both gallbladder function and anatomy (34).

Very few gallstones are visible in magnetic resonance images, and those that are seen usually contain clefts or pores (21). MR is fairly sensitive to cholecystitis because edema prolongs the T_1 of the gallbladder wall and surrounding liver parenchyma (**Figure 8-25**). MR has detected some cases of cholecystitis missed by ultrasound (19). In one case ultrasound suggested cholecystitis while MR clearly showed a large empyema of the gallbladder (22).

Pancreas

The posterior aspect of the pancreas is delineated well by the splenic vein (**Figure 8-26**). The anterior aspect of the pancreas may be partly or completely outlined by fat; however, both fat and pancreatic tissue have short T_1 values and can be difficult to distinguish (23). Opacification of bowel with oral paramagnetic contrast agents may help outline the pancreas in a few cases. Pancreatic carcinoma and pancreatitis both have prolonged T_1 values, and in these cases the pancreas may be difficult to separate from fluid-filled bowel loops that are dark unless a paramagnetic contrast medium is used. In many cases, pancreatitis, inflamed peri-pancreatic tissue, and carcinoma cannot be distinguished (24). Extension of carcinoma into the splenic vein and into other venous structures may be routinely visible, and MR may contribute to preoperative staging (17). In cases of common bile or pancreatic duct obstruction, the dilatation itself is often visible but obstructing stones usually are not (15). Pancreatic psuedocysts often can be identified by their typical T_1 and T_2 values (15) (**Figure 8-27**). Improved characterization of peripancreatic fluid collections and pseudocyst contents may be possible. A major current limitation in pancreatic imaging is reduced image quality because of respiratory motion (24).

Kidneys

The kidneys and liver have similar T_1 values. The upper pole of the right kidney can be imaged separately from the liver by obtaining SE sequences in the sagittal plane (25). The renal cortex and medulla are better distinguished by MR than by other imaging modalities (**Figure 8-28**). Changes in their appearance have been observed with increased hydration in normal subjects, presumably because of increased plasma volume in the cortex and increased urine in the collecting tubules of the medulla (25). Loss of the normal distinction between cortex and medulla occurs in chronic glomerulonephritis (23).

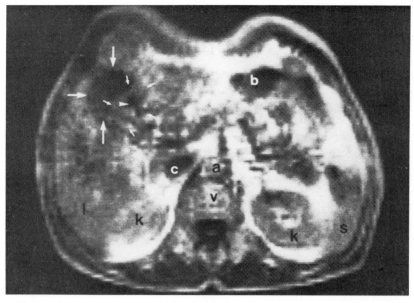

A

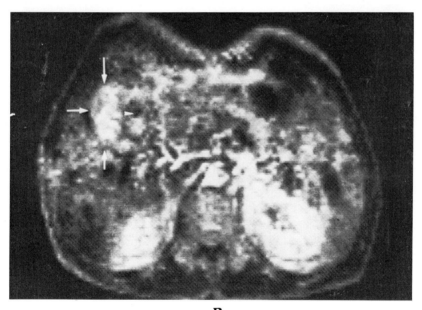

B

Figure 8-25. Periocholecystic abscess: SE. A, the abscess (large arrows) has low intensity in the short TR/moderate TE image. The gallbladder wall is indicated by small arrows. **B,** the abscess has high intensity in the long TR/moderate TE images because of prolonged T_2 and reduced T_1 weighting with this sequence. A gallstone (arrowhead) yields no signal in either image. (Reprinted with permission from Rupp, N., Reiser, M., and Stetter, E.: The diagnostic value of morphology and relaxation times in NMR imaging of the body. Eur. J. Radiol. 3:68-76, 1983.)

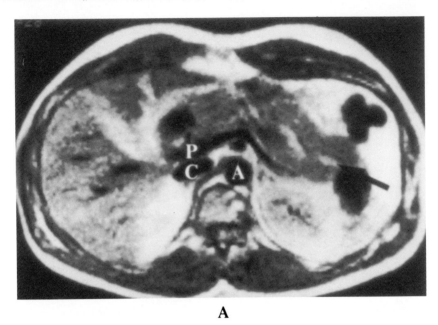

A

B

Figure 8-26. Normal pancreas: SE. A, the posterior aspect of the pancreas is clearly outlined by the portal vein (P). The anterior aspect of the pancreatic body and tail are separated from the collapsed stomach by adipose tissue (arrow). Bowel and pancreas have similar intensity in some images, and contrast administration may be necessary to distinguish them. C = vena cava; A = aorta. **B,** the size, shape, and intensity of the stomach changes when distended with air and water. (Reprinted with permission from Stark, D.D., and others: Magnetic resonance and CT of the normal and diseased pancreas; a comparative study. Radiology 150:153-162, 1984.)

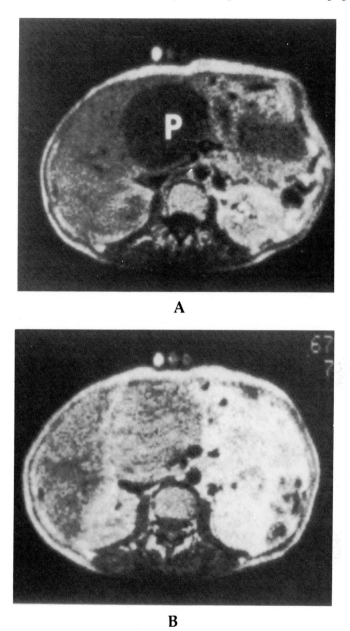

A

B

Figure 8-27. Pancreatic pseudocyst: SE. A, the pseudocyst (P) has very low intensity in the short TR/short TE image because of a very long T_1. **B,** the intensity of the pseudocyst is greater in the long TR/long TE image because of the very long T_2 of the pseudocyst fluid. (Reprinted with permission from Margulis, A.R.: Overview; current status of clinical magnetic resonance imaging. Radiographics 4:76-96, 1984.)

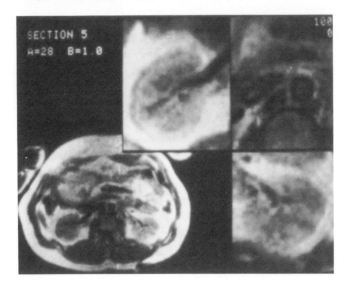

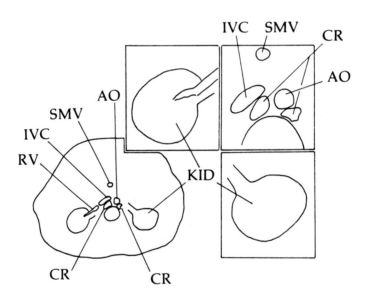

Figure 8-28. Normal kidney: SE. The renal cortex, medulla, and renal vein (RV) are all clearly seen in the normal and enlarged MR images. Also visible are the aorta (AO), superior mesenteric vein (SMV), inferior vena cava (IVC), and diaphragmatic crura (CR). (Reprinted with permission from Crooks, L., and others: Nuclear magnetic resonance whole body imager operating at 3.5 KGauss. Radiology 143:169-174, 1982.)

MR is useful in evaluating urinary obstruction and differentiating it from reflux. In obstruction the parenchyma is outlined on one side by urine and on the other side by perinephric fat, so that the degree of cortical thinning is easily assessed (25). Although both reflux and obstruction are characterized by a dilated renal pelvis, they can be distinguished because the distinction between cortex and medulla is lost in obstruction but not in reflux (25) (**Figure 8-29**). MR could prove useful in the evaluation of renal transplants because it can exclude obstruction and because the degree of T_1 prolongation in the kidney appears to correlate with the severity of rejection (25). However, it is unknown whether acute tubular necrosis can be differentiated from acute rejection by proton imaging.

The intravenous pyelogram will probably remain the primary screening test for renal disease. Following intravenous pyelography, MR may become the modality of choice in the evaluation of renal masses because it accurately differentiates simple cysts from solid masses, can frequently differentiate carcinoma from other tumors, shows extension of carcinoma through the renal capsule, and can reveal invasion of the intrarenal veins and the IVC (26) (**Figures 8-30** and **8-31**). MR can sometimes characterize the fluid content of cystic masses such as hemorrhage, serous fluid, necrosis, or purulent material (27); however, further experience is needed to define T_1 and T_2 values that are specific for different cystic fluids.

Normal adrenals can be seen in many cases. They are usually well outlined by fat; however, when the right adrenal is juxtaposed to the liver, distinction between the two can be difficult. The adrenal cortex and medulla can be distinguished (27), and this distinction may assist in the differentiation of adrenal tumors, adenomas, and hyperplasia. The spatial resolution of MR may be inadequate to prove whether a small tumor arises within or adjacent to the adrenal; infiltration of the liver by adrenal tumors cannot always be ruled out (15).

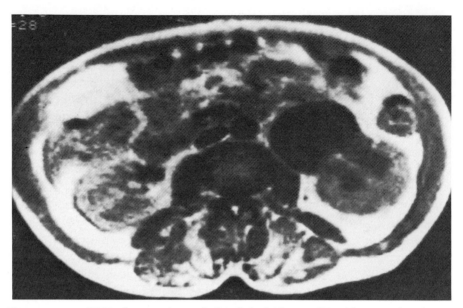

Figure 8-29. UPJ obstruction of the left kidney: SE. The renal pelvis is markedly dilated and dark because of the long T_1 of urine. The distinction between cortex and medulla is lost in obstruction, but not in reflux. (Reprinted with permission from Hricak, H., and others: Nuclear magnetic resonance imaging of the kidney. Radiology 146:425-432, 1983.)

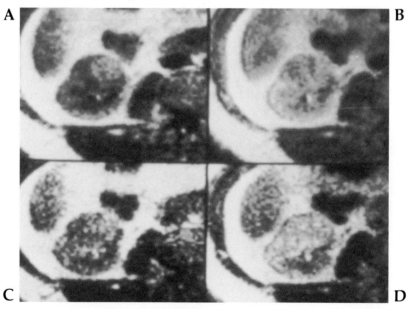

Figure 8-30. Renal cell carcinoma: SE. A, in the short TR/short TE image this tumor is nearly isointense with normal cortex. It is surrounded by a low intensity band of tissue proven to be a tumor pseudocapsule at pathology. The pseudocapsule is not demonstrated as well with other pulse intervals: **B,** moderate TR/short TE; **C,** short TR/moderate TE; and **D,** moderate TR/moderate TE. (Reprinted with permission from Hricak, H., and others: Nuclear magnetic resonance imaging of the kidney; renal masses. Radiology 147:765-772, 1983.)

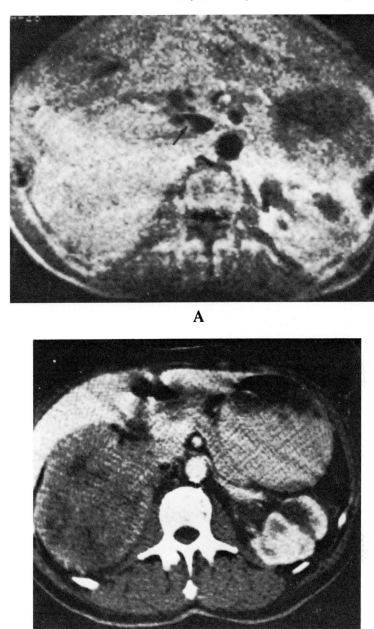

A

B

Figure 8-31. Renal cell carcinoma. A, SE; B, contrast-enhanced CT. The magnetic resonance image shows a nodular mass (arrow) within the lumen of the inferior vena cava. This mass subsequently was proven surgically to be tumor extension. The presence or absence of tumor in the inferior vena cava frequently cannot be determined with CT. (Reprinted with permission from Hricak, H., and others: Nuclear magnetic resonance imaging of the kidney; renal masses. Radiology 147:765-772, 1983.)

Pelvis

Magnetic resonance imaging of the pelvis is not degraded significantly by respiratory motion. The contrast among normal solid tissues is increased by the presence of fat, fluid, and gas. The flexibility of multiplanar imaging assists in the demonstration of normal anatomy and the extent of tumor invasion. The perineal muscles and the base and dome of the bladder are visualized best in sagittal and coronal sections, and the bladder, uterus, and rectum are easy to distinguish. Other normal structures visible in routine images include the urogenital diaphragm, levator ani muscles, ligaments, the cervix, ovaries, testes, prostate, and seminal vesicles (28, 29) (**Figure 8-32** and **8-33**). Although the contrast from flowing blood distinguishes vessels from adjacent lymph nodes and helps identify adenopathy, small abnormal lymph nodes cannot always be distinguished from other structures.

The T_1 and T_2 values of the normal prostate are similar to those for benign prostatic hypertrophy, whereas prostatic carcinoma may have nodules with prolonged T_1 and T_2 values leading to an inhomogeneous appearance in the image (**Figure 8-34**). It is not yet known whether benign hypertrophy, prostatitis, and prostatic carcinoma can be reliably distinguished. A 1-cm carcinoma of the prostate has been detected **in situ** (30), and invasion of the bladder base and pelvic fat by more advanced tumors can be demonstrated. Some tumor deposits not seen at surgery or with CT have been detected (28) with MR, and this modality probably is more accurate than CT in staging both prostatic and transitional cell carcinomas (29, 31) (**Figure 8-35**).

The myometrium and endometrial layers of the uterus can be distinguished in images that accentuate differences in T_2 (**Figure 8-36**). Variations have been observed in the morphology of the endometrium before, during, and after menarche, as well as changes in the thickness during the menstrual cycle (29). Both uterine leiomyomas and deposits of endometriosis can be seen; however, these conditions apparently do not have a characteristic appearance in MR (28, 29).

The normal ovary can be distinguished from surrounding fat in images that accentuate T_1 differences. Various appearances have been observed for cysts, and there is not yet enough experience to correlate size and image intensity with specific types of cysts. Although dermoid cysts are often intense because of their high fat content (**Figure 8-37**), they may be dark if they contain serous fluid (28).

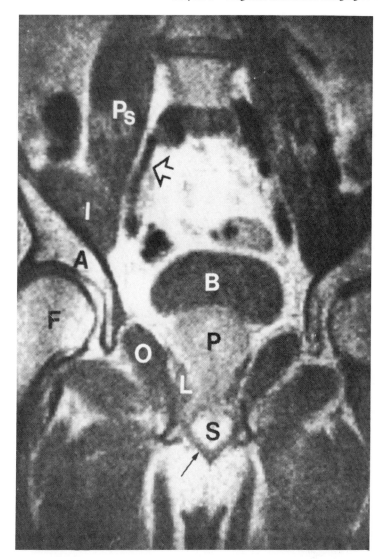

Figure 8-32. Normal pelvis: coronal SE. The levator ani muscle (L) is separated by fat from the obturator internus muscle (O) and the base of the prostate gland (P). The prostate gland indents the floor of the bladder (B). S = corpus spongiosum; F= femoral head; A = acetabulum; P_s = psoas major; I = iliacus; small arrow = bulbospongiosus; open arrow = common iliac vein. (Reprinted with permission from Hricak, H.: pelvis. In Margulis, A.R. and others, editors: Clinical Magnetic Resonance Imaging. San Francisco: 1983, Radiology Research and Education Foundation.)

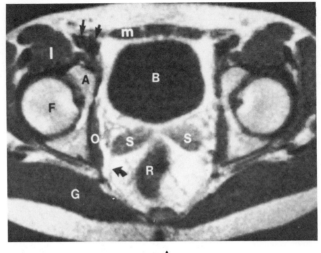

A

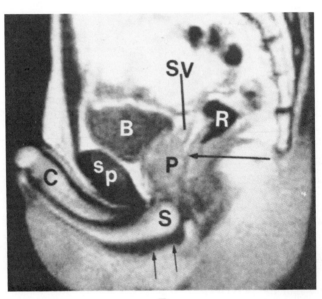

B

Figure 8-33. Normal male pelvis. A, transverse view; B, sagittal view. The bladder (B) has low intensity because it is filled with urine. Structures labelled in the transverse image are the seminal vesicles (S), the rectum (R), the femoral head (F), the acetabulum (A), the obturator internus muscle (O), the iliopsoas muscle (I), the rectus abdominis muscle (m), the gluteus maximus muscle (G), the vesicorectal fascia (curved arrow), and the femoral artery and vein (arrows). Structures labelled on the sagittal image: seminal vesicle (SV), corpus spongiosus (S), the bladder (B), the corpora cavernosa (C), the symphysis pubis (sp), the prostate gland (P), the rectum (R), the bulbospongiosus muscle (arrows), and the Denonvilliers fascia (long arrow) separating the prostate gland from the rectum. (Reprinted with permission from Hricak, H., and others: Anatomy and pathology of the male pelvis by magnetic resonance imaging. Am. J. Roentgenol. 141:1101-1110, 1983.)

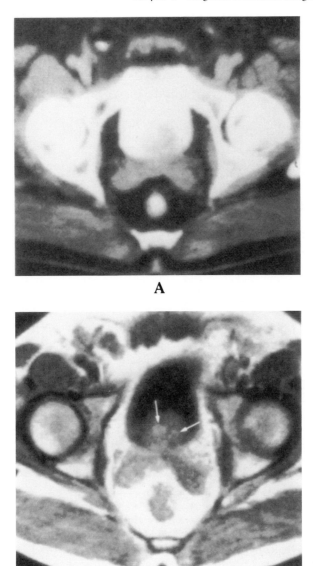

A

B

Figure 8-34. Prostatic carcinoma. A, CT; B, SE. A, the prostate gland in the CT image is enlarged and protrudes into the bladder lumen but has a homogeneous intensity. The seminal vesicles appear normal. **B,** the enlarged prostate protrudes into the bladder in the SE image but is inhomogeneous in intensity, with at least two areas of higher intensity (arrows). The right seminal vesicle is enlarged and has higher intensity produced by tumor invasion that subsequently was confirmed surgically. (Reprinted with permission from Hricak, H., and others: Anatomy and pathology of the male pelvis by magnetic resonance imaging. Am. J. Roentgenol. 141:1101-1110, 1983.)

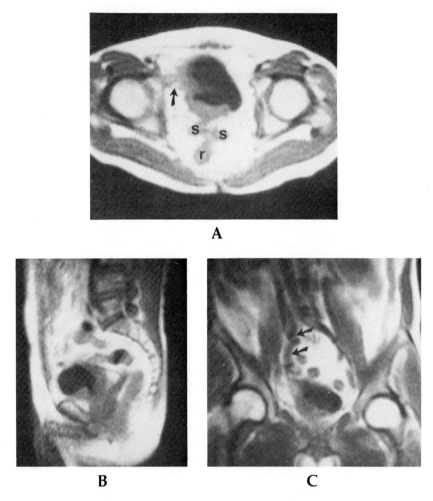

A

B **C**

Figure 8-35. Bladder carcinoma: SE. A, the transverse image shows irregular thickening of the bladder wall and extension into perivesical fat (arrow). At surgery, perivesical fat was thought to be free of tumor, but histological examination showed tumor infiltration. S = seminal vesicles; r = rectum. **B,** the sagittal image is best for evaluating the floor and dome of the bladder and shows the full extent of the tumor along the posterior wall. **C,** the coronal image shows obstruction of the right ureter (arrow) by tumor in the wall of the bladder. (Reprinted with permission from Bryan, P.J., and others: NMR scanning of the pelvis; initial experience with a 0.3T system. Am. J. Roentgenol. 141:1111-1118, 1983.)

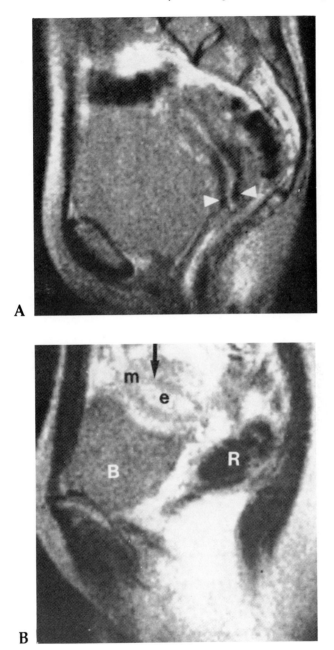

Figure 8-36. Normal female pelvis: SE. A, there is a high-intensity region, presumably blood, extending below the cervix into the posterior vagina during menstruation. The thin endometrium cannot be distinguished from the myometrium. There is clear distinction between the anterior and posterior cervical lips (arrows). **B,** in another patient, there is clear differentiation of the myometrium (m) and endometrium (e) in the secretory phase, with a low-intensity line separating the two (arrow). The bladder (B) and rectum (R) are also visible. (Reprinted with permission from Hricak, H., and others: Magnetic resonance imaging of the female pelvis; initial experience. Am. J. Roentgenol. 141:1119-1128, 1983.)

153

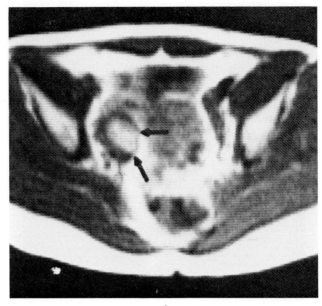

A

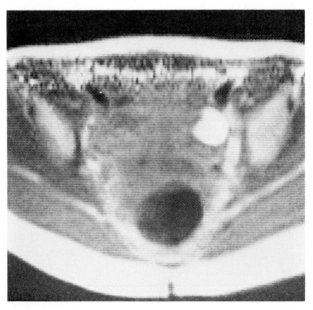

B

Figure 8-37. Follicular, A, and dermoid ovarian, B, cysts: SE. The follicular cyst (arrows) has moderately high intensity, presumably from prolonged T_2 and increased mobile proton density. It is surrounded by lower intensity ovarian tissue. The dermoid has very high intensity, presumably due to its fat content. (Reprinted with permission from Bryan P.J., and others: NMR scanning of the pelvis; initial experience with a 0.3T system. Am. J. Roentgenol. 141:1111-1118, 1983.)

Musculoskeletal System

Sagittal and coronal images are advantageous in demonstrating the extent of most types of bone pathology and are extremely useful in preoperative planning (15). Roentgenographic and CT images both reveal destruction better than does MR; however, areas where soft tissues have invaded bone and areas of cortical thinning can be appreciated better with MR (32). Magnetic resonance imaging is very sensitive to marrow replacement by benign tumors, metastases, and primary malignancies, and may be more accurate than either bone scans or CT in defining the extent of osteosarcoma (33). While CT and MR both show extraosseous tumor components, soft tissue abnormalities may appear more extensive with MR because of a decreased signal intensity in adjacent normal subcutaneous fat and bone marrow (33) (**Figure 8-38**). Aseptic necrosis and osteomyelitis produce areas of prolonged T_1 in the marrow, and MR is more sensitive than either plain films or CT in depicting these conditions.

The cruciate ligaments and menisci can be seen with MR, although applications of this capability have not yet been defined. MR may be useful in following patients with synovial inflammation if purulent, bloody, and serous synovial fluid collections can be differentiated (35). Other possible applications include venous thrombosis, muscular dystrophy (33), lower limb deformity in children (1), and evaluation of fractures when the extremity is casted (33).

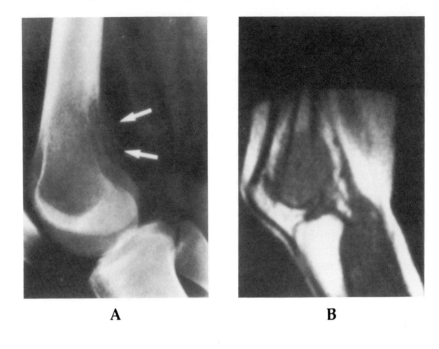

A   B

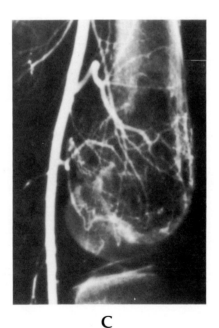

C

Figure 8-38. Osteosarcoma of the distal femur: A, lateral radiograph; B, sagittal PS; and C, angiogram. The radiograph demonstrates cortical bone destruction and a posterior soft tissue mass (arrows). The PS image reveals the extent of marrow replacement by tumor, posterior cortical bone destruction, and invasion of deep fat both anteriorly and posteriorly. The angiogram demonstrates abnormal tumor vessels in a distribution corresponding to the tumor seen on the PS image. (Reprinted with permission from Brady, T.J., and others: NMR imaging of leg tumors. Radiology 149:181-187, 1983.)

References

1. Smith, F.N.: The value of NMR imaging in pediatric practice: A preliminary report. Pediatr. Radiol. 13:141-147, 1983.

2. Crooks, L.E., Mills, C.M., and Davis, P.L.: Visualization of cerebral and vascular abnormalities by NMR imaging: Effects of imaging parameters on contrast. Radiology 144:843-852, 1982.

3. Gamsu, G., and others: Nuclear magnetic resonance imaging of the thorax. Radiology 147:473-480, 1983.

4. Cohen, A.M., and others: NMR evaluation of hilar and mediastinal lymphadenopathy, Radiology 148:739-742, 1983.

5. Higgins, C.B., and others: Nuclear magnetic resonance imaging of the cardiovascular system. Radiographics 4:122-136, 1984.

6. Fletcher, B.D., and others: Gated magnetic resonance imaging of congenital cardiac malformation. Radiology 150:137-140, 1984.

7. Buonanno, F.: Clinical applications of nuclear magnetic resonance (NMR). Disease-a-Month 29:1-81, 1983.

8. Herfkens, R.J., and others: Nuclear magnetic resonance imaging of the cardiovascular system: Normal and pathologic findings. Radiology 147:749-759, 1983.

9. Herfkens, R.J., and others: Nuclear magnetic resonance imaging of the infarcted muscle: A rat model. Radiology 147:761-764, 1983.

10. Higgins, C.B., and others: Cardiovascular system. In Margulis, A.R., and others, editors: *Clinical Magnetic Resonance Imaging.* San Francisco: 1983, Radiology Research Education Foundation.

11. Kaufman, L., and others: The potential impact of nuclear magnetic resonance imaging on cardiovascular diagnosis. Circulation 67:251-257, 1983.

12. Herfkens, R.J., and others: Nuclear magnetic resonance imaging of atherosclerotic disease. Radiology 148:161-166, 1983.

13. Ross, R.J., and others: Nuclear magnetic resonance imaging and evaluation of human breast tissue: Pulmonary clinical trials. Radiology 143:195-205, 1982.

14. El Yousef, S.J., and others: Initial experiment with nuclear magnetic resonance (NMR) imaging of the human breast. J. Comput. Assist. Tomog. 7:215-218, 1983.

15. Rupp, N., Reiser, M., and Stetter, E.: The diagnostic value of morphology and relaxation times in NMR imaging of the body. Eur. J. Radiol. 3:68-76, 1983.

16. Borkowski, G.P., and others: Nuclear magnetic resonance (NMR) imaging in the evaluation of the liver: Preliminary experience. J. Comput. Assist. Tomog. 7:768-784, 1983.

17. Higgins, C.B., and others: Nuclear magnetic resonance imaging of vasculature of abdominal viscera: Normal and pathologic features. Am. J. Roentgenol. 140:1217-1225, 1983.

18. Margulis, A.R., and others: Nuclear magnetic resonance in the diagnosis of tumors of the liver. Sem. Roentg. 17:123-126, 1983.

19. Smith, F.W., and others: Nuclear magnetic resonance tomographic imaging in liver disease. Lancet May 2, 1981, 963-966.

20. Doyle, F.H., and others: Nuclear magnetic resonance imaging of the liver: Initial experience. Am. J. Roentgenol. 138:193-200, 1982.

21. Moon, K.L., and others: Nuclear magnetic resonance imaging characteristics of gallstones in vivo. Radiology 148:753-756, 1983.

22. Pollet, J.E., and others: Whole-body nuclear magnetic resonance imaging: The first report of its use in surgical practice. Br. J. Surg. 68:493-494, 1981.

23. Henderson, R.G.: Nuclear magnetic resonance imaging: A review. J. Rox. Soc. Med. 76:206-212, 1983.

24. Stark, D.D., and others: Magnetic resonance and CT of the normal and diseased pancreas: A comparative study. Radiology 150:153-162, 1984.

25. London, D.A., and others: Nuclear magnetic resonance imaging of the kidney. Radiology 146:425-432, 1983.

26. Hricak, H., and others: Nuclear magnetic resonance imaging of the kidney: Renal masses. Radiology 147:765-772, 1983.

27. Moon, K.L., and others: Nuclear magnetic resonance imaging of the adrenal gland: A preliminary report. Radiology 147:155-160, 1983.

28. Bryan, P.J., and others: NMR scanning of the pelvis: Initial experience with a 0.3T system. Am. J. Roentgenol. 141:1111-1118, 1983.

29. Hricak, H., and others: Magnetic resonance imaging of the female pelvis: Initial experience. Am. J. Roentgenol. 141:1119-1128, 1983.

30. Davis, P.L.: *Clinical Applications of NMR.* Chicago: 1983, Society of Nuclear Medicine (Technologist Section).

31. Hricak, H., and others: Anatomy and pathology of the male pelvis by magnetic resonance imaging. Am. J. Roentgenol. 141:1101-1110, 1983.

32. Brady, T.J., and others: NMR imaging of leg tumors. Radiology 149:181-187, 1983.

33. Kean, D.M., and others: Nuclear magnetic resonance imaging of the knee: Examples of normal anatomy and pathology. Br. J. Radiol. 56:355-364, 1983.

34. Hricak, H., and others: Nuclear magnetic resonance imaging of the gallbladder. Radiology 147:481-484, 1983.

35. Moon, K.L., and others: Musculoskeletal applications of nuclear magnetic resonance. Radiology 147:161-171, 1983.

Chapter 9
Magnetic Resonance Spectroscopy

Introduction

Detecting the presence of certain compounds in tissue samples, measuring their concentration, and obtaining information about the chemical environment of cells has traditionally been the province of "freeze clamping" techniques. In freeze clamping, tissue samples are analyzed by routine chemical methods following quick freezing to prevent chemical breakdown. Under the best of circumstances, considerable information about a compound's intracellular chemical environment is lost with this technique; furthermore, the sample is destroyed during chemical extraction. Many duplicate specimens must be analyzed to generate statistically significant data, particularly for studies of changes in the samples occasioned by an experimental protocol. Each specimen may be subjected to a number of different analytical procedures, one for each compound. Freeze clamping studies cannot be used to assess rapid changes such as those occurring during a heart beat, since the freezing process alone may require a second or so for implementation.

Magnetic resonance spectroscopy is noninvasive, does not disturb cellular functioning, and provides minute-to-minute information about the tissue sample. Metabolic changes can be correlated with organ function during experimentally induced alterations in blood flow or the supply of essential metabolites. A single organ can be studied over an extended period, cause and effect relationships can be defined with regard to tissue damage, and recovery processes can be studied in detail.

Factors that regulate reaction rates **in vivo** often cannot be determined accurately **in vitro** with standard chemical techniques. The departure of certain reactions from equilibrium, the forward and backward rates of chemical reactions, and the dominant pathways of biosynthesis in tissue samples can all be measured by magnetic resonance "saturation transfer" experiments.

Technical Considerations

"Chemical shifts" (i.e., slight changes in resonance frequency of an element that reflect the structure of the chemical compound into which the element is incorporated) were demonstrated a few years after development of nuclear magnetic resonance. Chemical shifts arise because the cloud of electrons in a molecule (**Figure 9-1**) introduces local variations in the applied magnetic field. The nature of the variations depends on the types of atoms in the molecule and the chemical bonds between the atoms. For example, the three phosphorus atoms of adenosine triphosphate (ATP), a molecule important in cellular energetics, have different chemical environments (**Figure 9-2**) and resonate at three distinct frequencies. Chemical shifts are independent of magnetic field strength and are expressed as a frequency difference in parts per million (ppm) relative to a reference compound. The range of chemical shifts is different for each nuclear species; for example, 15 ppm for protons, 40 ppm for phosphorous-31, and 200 ppm for carbon-13.

An NMR spectrometer detects chemical shifts by measuring the energy absorbed from a series of radiofrequency pulses as a function of frequency. Every compound has a unique combination of chemical shifts and a characteristic spectrum of energy absorption. Hence, NMR can be used to detect the presence of quantity of a particular compound. The chemical structure of an unknown compound often can be determined from analysis of its energy absorption spectrum. NMR spectroscopy can be used to determine the concentration of a compound, since the area under a spectral absorption peak is proportional to the number of nuclei present in a particular chemical configuration, provided that full T_1 relaxation occurs between rf pulses. When pulses are repeated at intervals less than 5 T_1 or so, less energy is absorbed and the area under the peak is no longer representative of only the number of nuclei. The T_1s of cellular compounds may be a second or more, and pulses may need to be spaced several seconds apart to obtain quantitative results. This requirement may lead to unacceptably long measurement times. Often all that is needed in an experiment is a percent change in concentration; in this circumstance, pulse spacing is not critical. The absolute concentration of a compound can be obtained by calibrating the sample against a solution of known concentration, or by routine chemical analysis.

Large molecules, and small molecules tightly bound to large molecules, have a short T_2 and do not form sharp NMR absorption peaks. This behavior is advantageous in the sense that only the "free" or metabolically available concentrations of metabolites are measured by NMR. It also simplifies the interpretation of NMR spectra since the number of detectable compounds is limited. However, many molecules and intracellular regions cannot be probed. For example, the signal

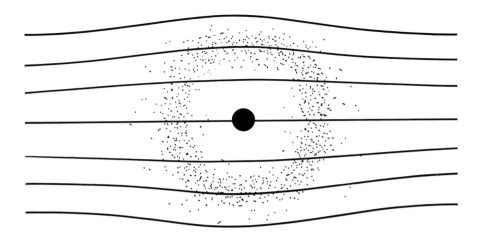

Figure 9-1. The electron cloud around a nucleus partially shields it from the magnetic field and alters its resonance frequency (chemical shift) by an amount that depends on the chemical identity of its neighbors and the type of bonds between them.

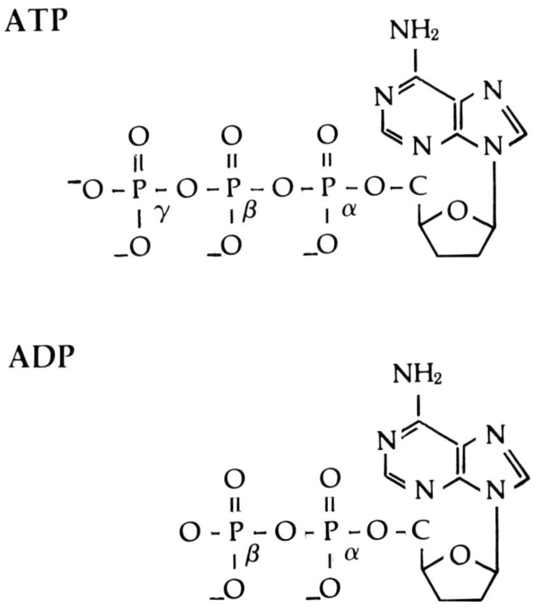

ATP

ADP

Figure 9-2. The chemical structure of ATP and ADP. The γ phosphorus of ATP and β phosphorus of ADP have nearly identical chemical environments and chemical shifts because each is bonded to four oxygen atoms and has a single phosphate group as its neighbor. The α phosphorus of ATP and α phosphorus of ADP also have the same chemical environment and chemical shift but differ from the terminal phosphorus nuclei. The chemical shift of the middle ATP (β) phosphorus nucleus is unique.

from the whole of the adrenal medulla comes from only a few compounds within chromaffin granules in the cell cytoplasm (1). In some instances the spatial selectivity of NMR can yield important information about the distribution of molecules in a cell. This information is difficult to determine by other means and can lead to distinction of intracellular and extracellular pools of metabolites.

When the compound is exposed to rf pulses at the frequency of a resonance peak, specific nuclei in the molecule absorb energy. A pulse of the proper intensity will equalize the distribution of nuclei into spin "up" and spin "down" energy states, causing the spectral peak to disappear. This condition is termed saturation. When some of the molecules are transformed by chemical reactions, their degree of saturation is transferred to the new molecules. The transfer alters the spectrum of the reaction product and allows the reaction rate to be determined. "Saturation transfer" NMR methods are restricted to reaction rates within a limited range; even with this limitation, however, they have led to a better understanding of metabolic pathways and physiologic activities.

Individual organs of living animals can be studied only by techniques that provide some spatial selectivity. One method is the "sensitive volume" technique (also called topical magnetic resonance or TMR). In this technique, the magnetic field is homogeneous over only a small "sensitive volume" at the center of the magnet bore. Over the remainder of the volume the field is inhomogeneous, and the signal is lost. Limiting the sensitive volume in this manner decreases the S/N ratio and increases the measurement time. Different organs can be examined by moving the animal inside the magnet bore so that the sensitive volume scans across the anatomy of interest. One design for moving the sensitive volume uses three orthogonal oscillating magnetic fields. The magnetic field is constant only in one small nodal volume, and this volume can be moved by changing the phase relationships of the oscillating fields. With this approach, the magnetic field is too inhomogeneous in the sensitive volume to yield maximum spatial resolution.

Another approach to TMR is to place rf generating coils on the skin surface. These coils are referred to as surface coils. The volume irradiated by a surface coil is approximately a hemisphere with a diameter equal to the coil diameter. Surface coil techniques are especially suited to examination of muscle, brain, and other rather superficial structures. They are less useful for studies of the liver, heart, and other deeper tissues because signals from these tissues are masked by those from more superficial structures. For example, several compounds can be detected by placing a surface coil over the liver. Sugar phosphate and inorganic phosphate resonances arise within muscle and blood as well as the liver. ATP resonances come from the liver and muscle, and phosphocreatinine resonance arises exclusively from muscle (2). Surface coils are especially useful for studying the brain; this organ is so sensitive to oxygen or blood deprivation that significant metabolic changes may occur even during rapid freezing in the freeze clamping technique.

A number of different nuclei can be observed by NMR spectroscopy. However, only three are present in sufficient concentration and yield a signal per nucleus that is intense enough for routine tissue studies. These three nuclei are hydrogen, carbon-13 (^{13}C), and phosphorus (^{31}P). Biological molecules contain many protons with similar chemical shifts; hence, proton spectra are often difficult, if not impossible, to analyze. Several experiments with ^{13}C and ^{31}P are presented in the following sections to illustrate the versatility of magnetic resonance spectroscopy.

Carbon-13

Carbon-13 spectroscopy competes with ^{14}C-labeled studies in which radioactive carbon-14 is incorporated at specific locations in a molecule. Carbon-14 compounds can be administered to cell extracts, bacteria, cell cultures, or animals, and samples can be subsequently withdrawn for radiochemical analysis. The incorporation of carbon-14 atoms into compounds within the samples yields information about metabolic pathways. However, these experiments can be complex, time consuming, and expensive.

A wide range of carbon compounds can be studied by NMR. Carbon-13 resonance peaks are sharply defined and cover a wide range of chemical shifts so that the resolution is excellent. The major limitation of ^{13}C spectroscopy is the low natural abundance of ^{13}C (only 1.1% of all carbon atoms are ^{13}C, and ^{12}C is not detectable by NMR because there are no unpaired protons or neutrons in the ^{12}C nucleus). Hence most NMR studies use ^{13}C enriched compounds. Without enrichment, ^{13}C NMR can detect glycogen (the depot form of glucose in muscle and liver), triglycerides, certain mobile lipids in membranes and a few other compounds (3). Although NMR could be used to measure concentrations of lipids throughout the body, the clinical usefulness of such measurements is unclear. One difficulty with non-enriched ^{13}C spectroscopy is that the signal from triglycerides and other lipids masks signals from more interesting compounds. Isopentane extraction of fat from human muscle samples has revealed differences between normal individuals and patients with muscular dystrophy and neurogenic muscle weakness (4).

Some elegant studies of the metabolism of rat livers have been performed with ^{13}C-enriched compounds (5-7). Details of the pathway by which labeled glycerol and alanine are incorporated into glycogen have been determined **in vivo**. Carbon-13 spectra revealed that the label appeared in several new compounds and in new positions in alanine and glucose molecules. Differences were found between the metabolism of liver cells in normal and hyperthyroid animals. The metabolism of glucose in different bacterial strains has been examined, revealing that certain reactions are preferred in different strains (8). However, clinical applications for such studies have not yet been identified. One limitation is that the cost of ^{13}C enriched compounds may be prohibitive for human studies.

Phosphorus-31

All phosphorus atoms in the body are ^{31}P. The signal intensity per nucleus is large for this element even in comparison to hydrogen. Phosphorus-31 spectra are simple to interpret. The phosphorus nuclei of DNA, RNA, most phospholipids, phosphoproteins, and bone are immobile and do not yield a measurable signal. Adenosine triphosphate (ATP), adenosine diphosphate (ADP), phosphocreatine (PCr), inorganic phosphate (P_i), and sugar phosphates are the principal mobile compounds present in sufficient concentrations in tissue to yield a measurable spectroscopic signal.

ATP is an energy-rich compound; it is degraded into adenosine diphosphate and inorganic phosphate with the release of energy:

$$ATP \rightleftharpoons ADP + P_i + Energy \qquad (1)$$

This reaction is essential to many processes that require energy, including muscle contraction, transport of chemicals and ions, and synthesis of large molecules. ATP can be resynthesized from ADP and P_i by utilization of energy from glucose metabolism. The resynthesis process is most efficient when oxygen is available (i.e., aerobic metabolism). ATP can be produced from glucose under anaerobic conditions, but the process is much less efficient and yields lactic acid, a toxic byproduct.

Phosphocreatine is also used to store energy and is particularly important in muscle cells. This compound is used to generate ATP for muscle contraction by a reaction catalysed by the enzyme creatine kinase:

$$PCr + ADP \rightleftharpoons Cr + ATP \qquad (2)$$

(Creatine kinase also catalyses the reverse reaction, in which ATP is consumed and PCr is restored.) The net reaction (+2) during muscle contraction is:

$$PCr \rightleftharpoons Cr + P_i$$

As PCr stores are utilized for muscle contraction, the PCr level falls and the P_i level increases.

NMR can be used to measure the concentrations of all the phosphorus compounds described above. It also can measure the rate at which phosphoenergetic reactions occur. The ratio of the concentrations of PCr and P_i (the PCr/P_i ratio) is an indicator of energy metabolism; a decline in the PCr/P$_i$ ratio usually occurs parallel to a decline in tissue oxygen pressure. The total concentrations of ATP and PCr indicate the amount of stored energy available to the cell. Significant stores of ATP and PCr are required for cell viability.

A typical ^{31}P spectrum for muscle (**Figure 9-3**) contains three peaks from ATP. The gamma ATP peak corresponds to the terminal phosphorus atom of ATP, and the alpha peak corresponds to the phosphorus atom attached to the adenosine molecule. The gamma peak may also represent the terminal phosphorus atom of ADP; however, the concentration of mobile ADP usually is low enough that its contribution is negligible. The alpha peak usually contains a small contribution from ADP and nicotinamide adenine dinucleotide (NAD). Peaks from PCr and P$_i$ are also well resolved in a ^{31}P NMR spectrum (**Figure 9-3**). NMR measurements of these compounds **in vivo** reveal that the PCr/ATP ratio is much higher, and the concentrations of metabolically

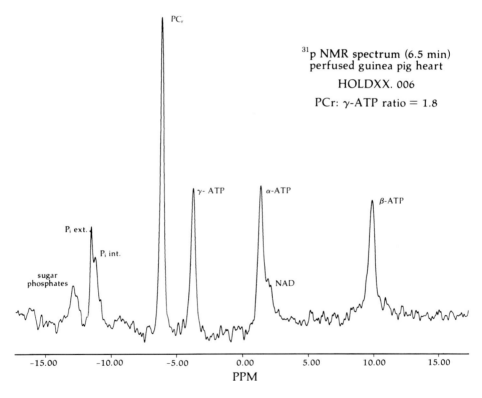

Figure 9-3. ^{31}**P spectrum of guinea pig cardiac muscle.** PCr, P$_i$, sugar phosphates, and the three ATP phosphorus nuclei have different chemical shifts and clearly resolved peaks. Analysis of the two components of the P$_i$ peak can be used to determine the intracellular-extracellular pH differences. (Reprinted with permission from Nunnally, R.L.: Localized measurements of metabolism by NMR methods: Some current and potential applications. In Witcofski, R.L., and others, editors: NMR Imaging. Winston-Salem, NC: 1981, Bowman-Gray School of Medicine.)

available ADP and P_i are much lower, than those measured by techniques such as freeze clamping. This discovery has raised the previous estimate of the energy potential available for cellular reactions by a factor of 10 to 20.

In many tissues there are two P_i peaks close together. The chemical shift of P_i depends on pH; hence the presence of more than one P_i peak implies the presence of regions of different pH. pH differences between the cell cytoplasm and mitochondria, bacteria and their growth media, and intracellular and extracellular compartments can be measured by NMR.

Potential applications of ^{31}P spectroscopy to clinical diagnosis are exciting. These applications could provide significant information about the normal functioning of organs and the metabolic response of these organs to injury and disease. Phosphorus-31 spectroscopy is particularly suited to the investigation of conditions that involve compromised blood flow (ischemia) and decreased availability of oxygen (hypoxia). Ischemia and hypoxia are involved in many pathological conditions, including myocardial infarction and stroke. Changes in cellular energy metabolism and pH should be detectable by ^{31}P spectroscopy before alterations appear in NMR images and long before abnormalities are detectible by either ultrasound or computed tomography. ^{31}P spectroscopy may be useful in determining the location, size, and extent of injury and in predicting the possibility of recovery. Spectroscopic measurement of ^{31}P should increase understanding of the mechanisms of ischemic cell damage and provide a method to assess therapeutic intervention.

Kidney

ATP, PCr, and P_i are visible in the NMR spectrum of the kidney, and measurements of changes in their concentrations have been used to assess the metabolic state of kidneys removed for transplantation (9, 10). At body temperature, ATP is nearly depleted 8 to 12 minutes after the kidney is surgically removed. When the kidney is chilled to 0°C and flushed with nonoxygenated media, however, ATP can be preserved for up to 6 hours. A precipitous drop in pH has been found to correlate with the point at which the kidney becomes nonfunctional; the time before the pH change occurs is longer at lower temperatures. This information is useful in determining the best way to preserve kidneys prior to transplantation. NMR may also be used to identify the optimum composition of flush solutions for kidney preservation.

Skeletal Muscle

ATP, PCr, P_i, and sugar phosphates can be observed in the spectra of skeletal muscle. Other peaks that probably represent phosphodiesters have been discovered and appear to be specific to different species and possibly also to muscle pathology (11). NMR measurements of the concentration of these compounds agree with results obtained by routine chemical analyses. The main difference between skeletal muscle and other tissues is that the PCr is highly concentrated in skeletal muscle. NMR has shown that ATP is chemically complexed with magnesium in the cell. Additional information provided by NMR includes the concentration of free ATP, the energy released by the breakdown of ATP to ADP in intact cells, the rate of lactic acid production, and the total rate of ATP turnover. Changes in the concentration of these metabolites have been monitored continuously in living muscles and correlated with the decline in contractile force and slowing of relaxation that occurs during muscle fatigue (12).

Gated NMR spectra have been obtained to correlate metabolic changes with different phases of muscle contraction. During contraction of normal muscle, the ATP concentration remains constant, indicating that ATP consumed in muscle contraction is regenerated very quickly either from stores of PCr or from breakdown of glucose (12). It appears that activation of enzymes to keep the store of PCr constant is closely associated with contraction rather than with an independent mechanism that senses a decline in the total amount of intracellular PCr (12). The enzymes may be activated by calcium released to initiate contraction (12).

Studies of muscle physiology during a series of contractions ending in muscle fatigue have shown that the force of contraction is proportional to the rate of ATP utilization (13). As ATP is regenerated, the fractions produced from stores of PCr and from glucose metabolism remain fixed (12).

During sustained muscle contraction, if the energy supply available for ATP generation is reduced by ischemia or hypoxia, pools of PCr are gradually depleted to maintain ATP levels. The breakdown of PCr produces increasing quantities of P_i, and anaerobic glucose metabolism produces lactic acid. Hence the concentration of P_i increases while the pH falls during anaerobic exercise. The PCr/P_i ratio is another measure of tissue oxygen delivery (14). Measurements of the PCr/P_i ratio and the pH may provide a noninvasive method for investigating normal exercise physiology. The reduction of blood flow in limbs from atherosclerosis or compartment syndromes may also be detectable by such methods (14).

A number of characteristic biochemical abnormalities have been identified in the different muscular dystrophies. NMR spectroscopy may assist in the differential diagnosis of these conditions and obviate the need for muscle biopsy. The concentration of glycerophosphorylcholine (GPC) can be measured by NMR; low values are found in Duchenne's dystrophy, and increased muscle levels are present in Werdnig-Hoffman syndrome (15). In McArdle's syndrome, genetic metabolic defects prevent ATP generation from the breakdown of glucose to lactic acid, and ischemic exercise leads to a small increase, rather than a decrease, in pH (16).

Cardiac Muscle

ATP, PCr, P_i, and sugar phosphate (probably glucose-6-phosphate) can be observed in the spectra of heart muscle. Hearts with infarcted regions also yield spectra with a broad peak that may represent calcium phophate precipitates in damaged cells (17). Data acquisition gated to the cardiac cycle has been used to evaluate variations in phosphoenergetics during contraction (18). The concentration of ATP and PCr are maximum when the heart is most relaxed, and minimum when aortic pressure is maximum. The concentration of P_i is 180° out of phase with those for ATP and PCr (18) (**Figure 9-4**). The ATP concentration falls steadily as the heart rate increases, while PCr levels remain constant and the P_i level increases slowly.

Within seconds after regions of heart muscle become ischemic, the force developed by contraction is decreased. In the next few minutes cellular changes can be observed with light microscopy, and after about 20 minutes the cells suffer irreversible damage (19). The relationship of the concentrations of ATP, PCr and P_i have been correlated with changes in cardiac function during ischemia and during recovery after restoration of normal blood flow. The concentration of ATP remains relatively constant during ischemia until stores of PCr are depleted (20); once blood flow resumes, the PCr can be resynthesized if the ischemic period is relatively short (21). The interrelationship of ATP and PCr pools is not clearly understood. Independent measurements of the reaction rates for creatine kinase in normal and ischemic heart muscle differ from those expected from changes in ATP and PCr concentrations (22). The implication is that the utilization of PCr to regenerate ATP, followed by ATP consumption in muscle contraction, is not a straightforward process. Further work is necessary to define the exact mechanisms involved.

In the study of heart disease, methods are needed to identify oxygen deficient regions of the muscle, the characteristics of the border between normal and damaged tissue, and the best methods to provide protection to ischemic regions (23). Ischemic heart muscle is characterized by high levels of lactic acid and a pH of 6.0 to 7.0 (24), with values at the lower end of this range more likely associated with irreversible damage (25). If the degree of ischemia is proportional to a decline in pH, it may be possible to identify ischemic regions by pH measurements.

Several compounds have been studied that protect heart muscle against ischemia. HEPES facilitates the recovery of ATP and PCr when ischemia is reversed (26, 27). Verapamil helps to maintain nearly nor-

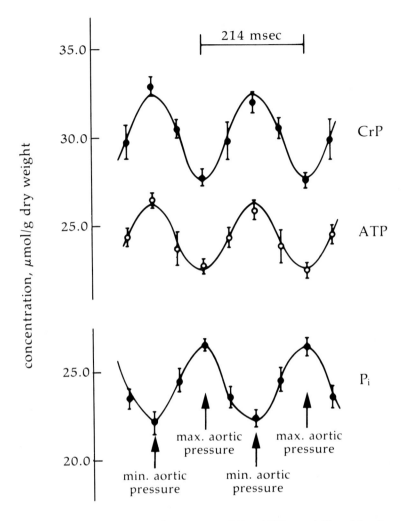

Figure 9-4. Concentration changes in PCr, ATP, and P_i with the cardiac cycle. Gated ^{31}P NMR data show that PCr (CrP) and ATP concentrations are highest when aortic pressure is minimum and lowest when aortic pressure is maximum. The concentration of P_i changes 180° out of phase with PCr and ATP concentrations. (Reprinted with modifications and permission from Fossell, E.T., and others: Measurement of changes in high energy phosphates in the cardiac cycle by using gated ^{31}P nuclear magnetic resonance. Proc. Nat. Acad. Sci. 77:3654-3658, 1980.)

mal levels of PCr and ATP in ischemic tissues because it is a coronary vasodilator and may protect mitochondria (17) (**Figure 9-5**). Chlorpromazine also preserves PCr and ATP although its effect is less dramatic (17). Administration of Inosine offers some protection because it can be metabolized to adenosine and phosphorylated to produce ATP (26, 28).

ATP is directly involved in muscle contraction and other vital biochemical reactions; hence, depletion of ATP stores is more significant than depletion of PCr stores during functional recovery in ischemia. P_i produced from PCr breakdown during ischemia appears to be preferentially shunted to PCr regeneration after reperfusion. This process impairs ATP resynthesis and may possibly prevent recovery (25). Identification of methods to modify P_i utilization may suggest new approaches to the treatment of myocardial infarction.

Brain

ATP, PCr, P_i, and sugar phosphates are also observed in brain tissue. An unexpected tentative identification of levels of ribose-5-phosphate, comparable to ATP levels was recently reported (29). Ribose-5-phosphate is a precursor in the synthesis of nucleic acids and is important in the biosynthesis of ATP, RNA and DNA but is not thought to be stored intracellularly. If confirmed, the finding of significant levels of ribose-5-phosphate raises fundamental questions about current understanding of brain biochemistry (29). In normal brain, the NMR-measured PCr/ATP ratio is higher than expected from data obtained by freezing studies, and the mobile ADP and P_i concentrations are much lower (16).

Ischemia of cerebral tissue produces functional changes within seconds and microscopic changes and irreversible damage in a few minutes. Very early stages of ischemia are difficult to study by NMR since observation usually requires at least a few minutes. Significant cerebral dysfunction may be present in mild hypoxia and hypoglycemia without any apparent energy deficit; hence changes may not be detected by NMR until consciousness is lost (30). These characteristics may cause problems in using NMR spectroscopy to define mechanisms of brain dysfunction and to determine the significance of cerebral insults.

Hypothermia of brain tissue during periods of ischemia has been found to greatly reduce the rate of decrease in intracellular pH. Although the PCr concentration falls as rapidly during hypothermia as when normal body temperature is maintained, ATP levels are preserved for at least 25 minutes at 0°C (19). Recovery of the normal metabolic state is possible following 20 minute periods of ischemia if hypothermia is utilized. The protective effect of hypothermia may be due to pH stabilization rather than to a reduction in metabolic requirements (19). Studies such as these may help refine techniques for protecting the brain during surgery.

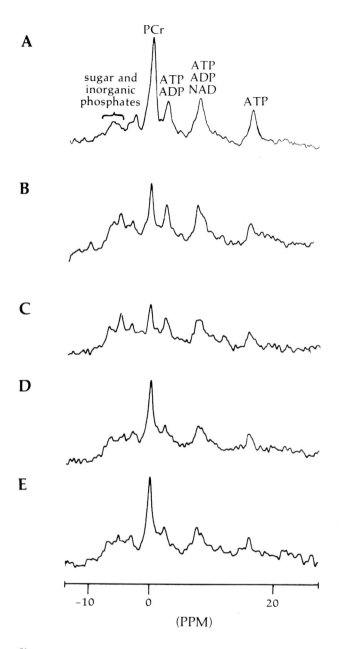

Figure 9-5. ^{31}**P spectra of cardiac muscle showing the effects of Verapamil treatment.** Chronological sequence of spectra obtained with a surface coil before and after Verapamil treatment in the regionally ischemic zone of a single heart. **A**, control spectrum; **B**, spectrum obtained betwen 5 and 30 minutes after left anterior descending coronary artery ligation; **C**, spectrum obtained between 30 and 55 minutes after ligation; **D**, the 5- to 30-minute interval after administration of Verapamil (60 to 85 minutes postligation); **E**, 30 to 55 minutes after the start of Verapamil treatment (85 to 110 minutes after ligation). (Reprinted with permission from Nunnally, R.L., and Bottomley, P.A.: Assessment of pharmacological treatment of myocardial infarction by phosphorus-31 NMR with surface coils. Science 211:177-180, 1981.)

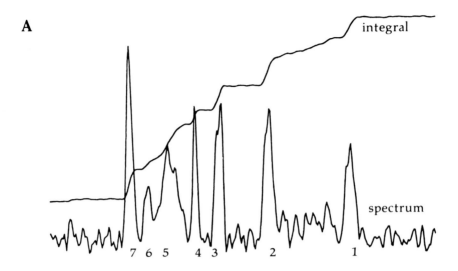

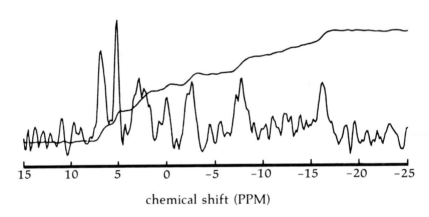

chemical shift (PPM)

Figure 9-6. ³¹P **spectra of brain in a normal infant, A, and in an infant with severe birth asphyxia and hypotonia, B.** Spectrum **A** is normal; and **B** has a very low PCr/P$_i$ ratio as determined from the ratio of the areas under the PCr and P$_i$ peaks. Infant **B** later developed porencephalic cysts. Peak assignments are as follows: 1 and 3 = ADP and magnesium complexed ATP; 2 = magnesium complexed ATP and NAD; 4 = PCr; 5= glycerol-3-phosphorylethanolamine and glycerol-3-phosphorylcholine; 6 = P$_i$; 7 = sugar phosphates (possibly ribose-5-phosphate). (Reprinted with permission from Cady, E.B. and others: Nonvasive investigation of cerebral metabolism in newborn infants by phosphorus magnetic resonance spectroscopy. Lancet 14:1059-1062, 1983.)

Several infants with severe intrapartum asphyxia or other gross neurological problems have been evaluated recently by NMR spectroscopy (29). In normal brain the PCr/P_i ratio was approximately 1.7. The PCr/P_i ratio of an infant with meningitis was reported as 0.7, suggesting moderately disordered cerebral metabolism. This infant had persistent hypotonia. A PCr/P_i ratio ranging from 0.2 to 1.0 has been observed in the first few days of life in asphyxiated infants. The ratio increased as the clinical condition of the patients improved. The infant with the lowest ratio later developed regions of porencephaly (**Figure 9-6**). No intracellular acidosis was found in asphyxia, presumably because excess lactic acid is removed by the circulatory system. This study concluded that ^{31}P NMR spectroscopy may be useful in detecting cerebral hypoxia in newborn infants in time to permit successful treatment.

Tumors

Metabolic studies of a number of malignant tumors have been conducted **in vitro** (31). In general, these tumors relied more heavily on anaerobic metabolism than do normal cells, and they exhibited higher levels of P_i. Levels of PCr and sugar phosphates were generally lower. No compound unique to a given tumor type was detected, but differences were observed in the balance between aerobic and anaerobic glucose metabolism. Tumors generally relied increasingly on anaerobic metabolism as they grew. The pH and PCr levels decreased, the P_i and sugar phosphates increased and ATP remained constant until the tumors became quite large. A shift toward aerobic metabolism was observed following chemotherapy, even before the mass of the tumor was reduced. The level of PCr was dramatically reduced in the acute stage following radiation treatment, while long-term radiation effects resembled those produced by chemotherapy. The authors suggest that identification of hypoxic areas in tumors could help to determine which tumors require administration of radiation sensitizers to achieve an optimal response to radiotherapy.

Chemical Shift Imaging

Technical difficulties in developing large bore magnets with stable and homogeneous magnetic fields of high intensity have been one of the major obstacles to the initiation of human studies by NMR spectroscopy. A prototype 1.5T magnet with a 1 meter bore has been used to obtain ^{31}P spectra from the human head by surface coils (**Figure 9-7**); the same unit can produce high-quality proton images (32). A major problem with surface coils is their rather coarse spatial selectivity. Magnetic resonance of protons and ^{31}P nuclei occurs at significantly different frequencies in the same magnetic field; hence hardware changes are necessary in switching from proton imaging to ^{31}P spec-

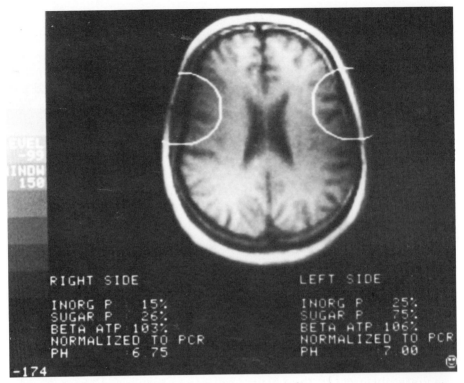

RIGHT SIDE   LEFT SIDE

INORG P   15%   INORG P   25%
SUGAR P   26%   SUGAR P   75%
BETA ATP   103%   BETA ATP   106%
NORMALIZED TO PCR   NORMALIZED TO PCR
PH   6.75   PH   7.00

-174

Figure 9-7. Normal brain: PS proton image and ^{31}P spectroscopic data. This represents the first spectroscopic study obtained with a whole body imager. (Courtesy of the General Electric Company.)

troscopy. This switching could require up to a few hours, during which the NMR system is unavailable for use.

Images of the spatial distribution of a metabolite can be obtained by mapping the intensity of its spectral peak. Images that reflect the concentration of PCr may be useful in detecting and evaluating stroke, and images based on pH may be helpful in studying myocardial infarction. Current proton imaging techniques cannot be applied to spectroscopic imaging because the magnetic field gradients destroy spectroscopic resolution. Chemical shift imaging techniques have been devised (33, 34) but they have not been applied **in vivo**. By far the major limitation of ^{31}P and ^{13}C chemical shift imaging is an unfavorable signal to noise ratio. In a reasonable length of imaging time, it may be possible to resolve only 20 or so volume elements within the region of interest (16).

References

1. Gadian, D.G., and Radda, G.K.: NMR studies of tissue metabolism. Ann. Rev. Biochem. 50:69-83, 1981.

2. Ackerman, J.J.H., and others: Mapping of metabolites in whole animals by ^{31}P NMR using surface coils. Nature 283:167-170, 1980.

3. Alger, J.R., and others: In vivo carbon-13 nuclear magnetic resonance studies of mammals. Science 214:660-662, 1981.

4. Barany, M., and others: Natural abundance ^{13}C NMR spectra of human muscle, normal and diseased. Mag. Res. Med. 1:30-43, 1984.

5. Cohen, S.M., and Shulman, R.G.: NMR Studies of gluconeogenesis in rat liver suspensions and perfused mouse livers. Phil. Trans. R. Soc. Lond. B. 289:407-411, 1980.

6. Cohen, S.M., Glynn, P., and Shulman, R.G.: ^{13}C NMR study of gluconeogenesis from labeled alanine in hepatocytes from euthyroid and hyperthyroid rats. Proc. Nat. Acad. Sci. 78:60-64, 1981.

7. Cohen, S.M., Ogawa, S., and Shulman, R.G.: NMR studies of gluconeogenesis in rat liver cells: Utilization of labeled glycerol in cells from euthyroid and hyperthyroid rats. Proc. Nat. Acad. Sci. 76:1603-1607, 1979.

8. Ugurbil, K., and others: High-resolution ^{13}C nuclear magnetic resonance studies of glucose metabolism in Eschemia *Coli*. Proc. Nat. Acad. Sci. 75:3742-3746, 1978.

9. Sehr, P.A., and others: Non-destructive measurements of metabolites and tissue pH in the kidney by ^{31}P nuclear magnetic resonance. Br. J. Exp. Path. 60:632-641, 1979.

10. Ackerman, J.J.H., and others: NMR studies of metabolism in perfused organs. Phil. Trans. R. Soc. Long. B. 289:425-436, 1980.

11. Meyer, R.A., and others: Application of ^{31}P NMR spectroscopy to the study of striated muscle metabolism. Am. J. Physiol. 242:1-11, 1982.

12. Dawson, M.J., Gadian, D.G., and Wilkie, D.R.: Studies of the biochemistry of contracting and relaxing muscles by the use of ^{31}P NMR in conjunction with other techniques. Phil. Trans. R. Soc. Lond. B. 289:445-455, 1980.

13. Dawson, M.J., Gadian, D.G., and Wilkie, D.R.: Mechanical relaxation rate and metabolism studied in fatiguing muscle by phosphorus nuclear magnetic resonance. J. Physiol. 299:465-484, 1980.

14. Shaw, D.: In vivo chemistry with NMR. In Kaufman, L., and others, editors: *Nuclear Magnetic Resonance Imaging in Medicine.* New York: 1981, Igaku-Shoin.

15. Burt, C.T., and others: Variations of phosphate metabolites in normal and Duchenne human muscle. Biophys. J. 21:184, 1978.

16. Gadian, D.G.: *Nuclear magnetic resonance and its application to living systems.* Oxford: 1982, Clarendon Press.

17. Nunnally, R.L., and Bottomley, P.A.: Assessment of pharmacological treatment of myocardial infarction by phosphorus-31 NMR with surface coils. Science 211:177-180, 1981.

18. Fossell, E.T., and others: Measurement of changes in high energy phosphates in the cardiac cycle by using gated ^{31}P nuclear magnetic resonance. Proc. Nat. Acad. Sci. 77:3654-3658, 1980.

19. Norwood, W.I., and others: Hypothermic circulatory arrest. J. Thorac. Cardio. Surg. 78:823-830, 1979.

20. Griffiths, J.R., and Iles, R.A.: Nuclear magnetic resonance—a magnetic eye on metabolism. Clin. Sci. 59:225-230, 1980.

21. Burt, C.T., and others: Analysis of intact tissue with ^{31}P NMR. Ann. Rev. Biophys. Bioeng. 8:1-25, 1979.

22. Hollis, D.P., and Nunnally, R.L.: Recent ^{31}P NMR studies of myocardium. Phil. Trans. R. Soc. Lond. B. 289:437-439, 1980.

23. Radda, G.K., and Seeley, P.G.: Recent studies on cellular metabolism by nuclear magnet resonance. Ann. Rev. Physiol. 41:749-769, 1979.

24. Gadian, D.G., and others: Phosphorus nuclear magnetic resonance studies on normoxic and ischemic cardiac tissue. Proc. Nat. Acad. Sci. 73:4446-4448, 1976.

25. Flaherty, J.P., and others: Mechanisms of ischemic myocardial cell damage assessed by phosphates 31 nuclear magnetic resonance. Circulation 65:561-571, 1983.

26. Ingwall, J.S.: Phosphorus nuclear magnetic resonance spectroscopy of cardiac and skeletal muscles. Am. J. Physiol. 242:729-744, 1982.

27. Manasche, P., and others: Nuclear magnetic resonance, a new method for noninvasive assessment of cardiac metabolism. Med. Progr. Technol. 8:183-185, 1982.

28. Ingwall, J.S., and others: ATP synthesis following anoxic in isolated profused rat hearts: Capacity of the salvage pathway. Circulation 60:11, 1979.

29. Cady, E.B., and others: Noninvasive investigation of cerebral metabolism in newborn infants by phosphorus magnetic resonance spectroscopy. Lancet, May 14:1059-1062, 1983.

30. Cox, D.W.G., and others: ^{31}P NMR studies on cerebral energy metabolism under conditions of hypoglycemia and hypoxia in vitro. Biochem. J. 212:365-370, 1983.

31. Ng, T.C., and others: ^{31}P NMR spectroscopy of in vivo tumors. J. Mag. Res. 49:271-286, 1982.

32. Bottomley, P.A., and others: Anatomy and metabolism of the normal brain studied by magnetic resonance at 1.5 Tesla. Radiology 150:441-446, 1984.

33. Brown, T.R., Kincaid, B.M., and Ugurbil, K.: NMR chemical shift imaging in three dimensions. Proc. Nat. Acad. Sci. 79:3523-3526, 1982.
34. Maudsley, A.A., and others: Spatially resolved high resolution spectroscopy by "Four Dimensional NMR." J. Mag. Res. 51-147, 1983.

Chapter 10
Current Status of MR Imaging

Magnetic resonance offers an approach to medical imaging that is significantly different from the imaging modalities heretofore available to the physician. Conventional imaging techniques such as radiography and fluoroscopy utilize the differential attenuation of x rays in the body to produce a pattern of shadows in the transmitted x-ray beam that can be captured by film or image intensifier. In nuclear medicine the distribution of radioactivity, and changes in its distribution with time, can be detected to reveal abnormalities in patient anatomy and physiology. Ultrasonic energy reflected from different interfaces within the body is used to construct ultrasound images of patient anatomy. Even though computed tomography is recognized today as a revolutionary tool introduced into medical imaging just over a decade ago, it still employs the differential attenuation of x rays as the fundamental tissue characteristic revealed in its images. Magnetic resonance imaging is decidedly different from all of these modalities and considerably more complex in its operation and in the interpretation of images. In large measure, this increased complexity constitutes both the promise and the challenge of MR. It also creates uncertainty in attempting to project the role MR ultimately will play in the arena of medical imaging.

Magnetic resonance imaging is different from its medical imaging predecessors because several tissue characteristics are accessible to imaging with this modality. Among these parameters are proton density, T_1 and T_2 relaxation rates, fluid flow, and spectral shifts of hydrogen and, ultimately, other elements. By selecting a particular imaging method (partial saturation, inversion recovery, spin-echo, etc.), these characteristics can be combined to yield images that emphasize one parameter over the other. Even within a single imaging method, the pulse sequences can be varied to yield images that differ significantly in their appearance. Both clinical experience and a fundamental understanding of the principles of magnetic resonance imaging are essential for accurate image interpretation.

Currently, considerable controversy reigns over the issue of the most desirable field strength for magnetic resonance imaging. Proponents of high field strength (1.0T and above) systems proclaim that

179

superior images are obtained because of improvements in the signal-to-noise ratio at the high field strengths. They also emphasize that higher field strengths are required for spectroscopy. Supporters of moderate field strength MR systems (0.15-0.5T) state that rf signals are attenuated at the higher frequencies associated with higher field strength MR units, creating difficulties in the imaging of deeper tissues. Furthermore, field uniformity may be difficult to maintain in magnets of higher field strength, and the fringe fields of stronger magnets extend over greater distances so that siting of the MR unit is more difficult, especially in an existing facility. Moderate field strength supporters point out that it may be impossible to design a machine that can shift quickly from imaging to spectroscopy. Unfortunately, experience at this time is inadequate to resolve many of these controversial issues.

Another unresolved issue is the role ultimately to be played by MR systems that employ permanent and resistive magnets. Because of their high consumption of electricity, units employing resistive magnets are confined at present to field strengths of 0.15T and below. These units require rather elaborate plumbing to accommodate flowing water used for cooling. Furthermore, images from resistive MR units are noisier and less esthetically pleasing than those from superconductive systems; whether they provide less diagnostic information is unresolved. They are significantly less expensive than superconductive systems and their reliability and performance have been good.

Permanent magnet units have many advantages. They produce no fringe magnetic fields and their siting is much easier. They have been constructed at field strengths up to 0.3T and conceivably could go higher. The weight of some permanent magnet units is great (e.g., 100 tons); however, new magnetic alloys permit a significant weight reduction. The purchase cost of a permanent magnet unit increases rapidly with field strength. At 0.3T, a permanent magnet unit costs more than a superconductive system of comparable field strength. Of course, there are no major continuing costs for cryogens or electricity with a permanent magnet system. Field nonuniformity and consequent image degradation appears to be a continuing problem with some permanent magnet units. Tunable pole pieces have been proposed to overcome this problem in some systems.

Another area of uncertainty is the degree to which precautions must be taken to shield an MR unit from its environment. Some installations have been built with structural iron noticeably absent and with meticulous attention to shielding against rf interference. Other installations have exercised considerably less caution in these areas, apparently without adverse effects. More information on the effectiveness of different approaches to siting design needs to be gathered to determine the degree of shielding required for a particular installation. Similarly, more data are needed on the effects of MR systems on pacemaker operation and on fetal development, as well as on other possible bioeffects of an MR examination.

Computer software controls all operational features of an MR unit, including the selection of pulse sequences and intervals and the display of the final image. Software differences among systems can be significant. The relative advantages of three-dimensional versus multiplanar imaging, the optimum method for measuring blood flow, the best sequences for demonstrating specific types of pathology, and the preferred reconstruction and image processing techniques are all areas of uncertainty at this time. Additional fundamental research and further clinical experience are needed to determine optimum software characteristics.

Software differences must be kept in mind when evaluating the results of clinical studies from different institutions. For example, initial MR studies of myocardial infarction were performed only with T_1 weighted pulse sequences (1). Demonstrable changes in infarcted myocardium were not detected until T_2 weighted imaging sequences were employed (2). No single group of investigators currently has equipment capable of utilizing the full range of pulse sequences and timing parameters available for magnetic resonance imaging. Specific pulse sequences helpful in revealing certain specific conditions may not be optimum at some centers. Equipment variations can also influence T_1 and T_2 measurements because these values depend on the magnetic field strength, the methods used to calculate T_1 and T_2, and on other characteristics that may vary from one MR unit to the next.

In spite of its infancy, MR already has some applications for which it may be the modality of choice. It appears to be superior to CT in evaluating a variety of central nervous system diseases. It is especially valuable in multiple sclerosis, diseases of the cervical spinal cord, posterior fossa lesions, and in patients who have a focal neurological examination and a normal CT study. MR has several advantages over CT in staging tumors of the head and neck, mediastinum, kidneys, and pelvis, and some advantages in evaluating the liver, spleen, pancreas, and skeletal system. It should prove useful in evaluating patients with surgical clips that degrade CT images. Gated cardiac studies are in the early stage of clinical evaluation and blood flow measurements are just being developed; both of these techniques show considerable promise. As clinical experience is accumulated, MR may well become the modality of choice in a number of other areas.

In many applications MR is extremely sensitive in detecting disease but sometimes does not yield a specific diagnosis; for example, tumors, inflammation, and infarctions can present identical appearances. Experience gained from interpretation of CT images has been very helpful even though CT and MR examine different tissue characteristics. The flexibility of MR may provide greater diagnostic specificity than CT, even though pathologic basis for changes in T_1 and T_2 is uncertain at this time. Extensive studies correlating MR appearance with lesion pathology are needed to understand the significance of lesion morphology and to refine imaging methods for specific lesions.

MR currently has several clinical limitations. Calcification and cortical bone pathology are not revealed well with MR. The evaluation of spinal degenerative diseases and trauma is limited by the similar appearance of spinal ligaments, osteophytes, intervertebral disc fragments, and cortical bone fragments, and by the spatial resolution and slice thicknesses available with current equipment. The pancreas sometimes cannot be distinguished from adjacent bowel loops, even in high-quality images, and respiratory motion often degrades images of the upper abdomen including the pancreas. Respiratory gating, improved spatial resolution, and contrast agents may ultimately circumvent some of these limitations.

Nonmagnetic alloys are used to fabricate most implantable metallic devices and these do not interact with the magnetic field. Patients with orthopedic prostheses, surgical clips, and wire sutures can usually be imaged safely. Compared to tissue, these objects absorb more rf energy, and there was concern initially that heating of large prostheses might be a problem for some patients (3). However, clinical experience has reduced this concern (4). In certain instances, rf energy absorption by metallic implants can interfere with imaging and produce localized image defects.

Magnetic field strength increases rapidly near the entrance to the bore of the MR magnet. In this region, magnetic objects experience a pull toward the center of the magnet. In the imaging volume, the field is homogeneous and magnetic objects experience a twisting force, or torque, as they try to align in the direction of the magnetic field. Neurological aneurysm clips, bridgework, and dental prostheses are often magnetic. Patients with aneurysm clips often cannot be examined with MR because the clips are attached to delicate tissues and could become dislodged in the magnetic field. Examination of patients with bridgework and dental prostheses is not contraindicated since these devices are not attached to critical tissues. However, magnetic objects in the imaging volumes may produce magnetic field distortions and significant image defects.

The most important issue related to magnetic resonance imaging is the question of what it will contribute ultimately to patient care. There is little question that exquisite images of the brain, spinal cord, pelvic anatomy, and certain other structures are provided by MR. Whether these exquisite images provide information that is not accessible by other means, and whether the information contributes in a meaningful way to patient diagnosis and treatment, remain to be determined. This determination is awaited by individuals and by agencies involved in efficacy evaluations, not the least of which is the Food and Drug Administration of the U.S. Department of Health and Human Services, the federal agency responsible for approving MR units for commercial distribution. Of equal importance are the Health Care Finance Administration (the federal agency responsible for administering the Medicare program) and various third-party insurance carriers who are awaiting proof of the clinical efficiency and cost effectiveness of MR before embarking on a cost reimbursement course for MR examinations.

Magnetic resonance is one of the most exciting and challenging imaging modalities to emerge in the history of medical imaging. At this time, it is impossible to evaluate its ultimate role in the clinical care of patients. In part this role will be determined by how well imaging specialists assimilate the fundamentals of magnetic resonance and apply them to the clinical arena in an efficient and cost-effective manner.

References

1. Buonanno, F.S., and others: Proton NMR imaging in experimental ischemic infarction. Stroke 14:178-184, 1983.

2. Higgins, C.B.: Imaging the heart with magnetic resonance. Diagn. Imag. 39-45, December 1983.

3. New, P.F.J., and others: Potential hazards and artifacts of ferromagnetic and nonferromagnetic surgical and dental devices in nuclear magnetic resonance imaging. Radiology 147:139-148, 1983.

4. Pavlicek, M.S.: Safety features about magnetic resonance units. NMR Update Series 1(2):2-14. Princeton: 1984, Continuing Professional Education Center, Inc.

Glossary
of MR Terms

(Reprinted with permission from the American College of Radiology. This glossary was prepared under the auspices of the subcommittee on MR nomenclature, within the MR committee on Imaging Technology and Equipment, ACR Commission on Magnetic Resonance, Thomas F. Meaney, M.D., Chairman.)

Acquisition time—see Image acquisition time.

ADC—see Analog to digital converter.

Adiabatic fast passage (AFP)—technique of producing rotation of the *macroscopic magnetization vector* by sweeping the *frequency* of an irradiating *RF* wave (or the strength of the *magnetic field*) through *resonance* (the *Larmor frequency*) in a time short compared to the *relaxation times*. Particularly used for *inversion* of the *spins*. A *continuous wave NMR* technique.

Adiabatic rapid passage—see Adiabatic fast passage.

AFP—see Adiabatic fast passage.

Analog to digital converter (ADC)—part of the *interface* that converts ordinary (analog) voltages, such as the detected *NMR signal,* into digital number form, that can be read by the *computer.*

Angular frequency (ω)—*frequency* of oscillation or rotation (measured, e.g., in radians/second) commonly designated by the Greek letter ω: $\omega = 2\pi f$, where f is frequency (e.g., in *hertz* (Hz)).

Angular momentum—a *vector* quantity given by the vector product of the momentum of a particle and its position vector. In the absence of external forces, the angular momentum remains constant, with the result that any rotating body tends to maintain the same axis of rotation. When a *torque* is applied to a rotating body, the resulting change in angular momentum results in *precession*. Atomic nuclei possess an intrinsic angular momentum referred to as *spin,* measured in multiples of Planck's constant.

185

Antenna—device to send or receive electromagnetic radiation. Electromagnetic radiation per se is not relevant to NMR, as it is the magnetic vector alone that couples the *spins* and the *coils,* and the term coil should be used instead.

Array processor—optional component of *computer* system specially designed to speed up numerical calculations like those needed in *NMR imaging.*

Artifacts—false features in the image produced by the imaging process.

B₀—a conventional symbol for the constant *magnetic (induction) field* in an *NMR* system. (Although historically used, H_O (units of *magnetic field* strength, ampere/meter) should be distinguished from the more appropriate B_O (units of magnetic induction, tesla).)

B₁—a conventional symbol for the *radiofrequency magnetic induction field* used in an *NMR* system (another symbol historically used is H_1). It is useful to consider it as composed of two oppositely rotating *vectors,* usually in a plane transverse to B_0. At the *Larmor frequency,* the vector rotating in the same direction as the *precessing* spins will interact strongly with the *spins.*

Bloch equations—phenomenological "classical" equations of motion for the *macroscopic magnetization vector.* They include the effects of *precession* about the *magnetic field* (static and *RF*) and the *T1* and *T2 relaxation times.*

Boltzmann distribution—if a system of particles which are able to exchange energy in collisions is in thermal equilibrium, then the relative number of particles, N_1 and N_2, in two particular energy states with corresponding energies, E_1 and E_2, is given by

$$\frac{N_1}{N_2} = \exp\left[-(E_1 - E_2)/kT\right]$$

where k is Boltzmann's constant and T is absolute temperature. For example, in *NMR* of protons at room temperature in a *magnetic field* of 0.25 *tesla,* the difference in numbers of *spins* aligned with the magnetic field and against the field is about one part in a million; the small excess of nuclei in the lower energy state is the basis of the net *magnetization* and the *resonance* phenomenon.

Carr-Purcell (CP) sequence—sequence of a *90° RF pulse* followed by repeated *180° RF pulses* to produce a train of *spin echoes;* useful for measuring *T2.*

Carr-Purcell-Meiboom-Gill (CPMG) sequence—modification of *Carr-Purcell RF pulse* sequence with 90° *phase* shift in the *rotating frame of reference* between the *90° pulse* and the subsequent *180° pulses* to reduce accumulating effects of imperfections in the 180° pulses. Suppression of effects of pulse error accumulation can alternatively be achieved by alternating phases of the 180° pulses by 180°.

Chemical shift (δ)—the change in the *Larmor frequency* of a given nucleus when bound in different sites in a molecule, due to the magnetic shielding effects of the electron orbitals. Chemical shifts make possible the differentiation of different molecular compounds and different sites within the molecules in high-resolution *NMR spectra.* The amount of the shift is proportional to *magnetic field* strength and is usually specified in parts per million (ppm) of the *resonance frequency* relative to a standard.

Coherence—maintenance of a constant *phase* relationship between rotating or oscillating waves or objects. Loss of phase coherence of the *spins* results in a decrease in the *transverse magnetization* and hence a decrease in the *NMR signal.*

Coil—single or multiple loops of wire (or other electrical conductor, such as tubing, etc.) designed either to produce a *magnetic field* from current flowing through the wire, or to detect a changing magnetic field by voltage induced in the wire.

Computer—as used for *NMR,* can be divided into central processing unit (CPU), consisting of instruction interpretation and arithmetic unit plus fast access memory, and peripheral devices such as bulk data storage and input and output devices (including, via the *interface,* the *spectrometer*). Under *software* control, the computer controls the *RF pulses* and *gradients* necessary to acquire data, and processes the data to produce *spectra* or images. (Note that devices such as the spectrometer may themselves incorporate small computers.)

Continuous wave NMR (CW)—a technique for studying *NMR* by continuously applying *RF* radiation to the sample and slowly sweeping either the RF *frequency* or the *magnetic field* through the *resonance* values; now largely superceded by *pulse NMR* techniques.

Contrast—contrast can be defined as the relative difference of the signal intensities in two adjacent regions. In a general sense, we can consider image contrast, where the strength of the image intensity in adjacent regions of the image is compared, or object contrast, where the relative values of a parameter affecting the image (such as *spin density* or *relaxa-*

tion time) in corresponding adjacent regions of the object are compared. If the two intensities are J_1 and J_2, a useful quantitative definition of contrast is $(J_1 - J_2)/(J_1 + J_2)$. Relating image contrast to object contrast is more difficult in *NMR imaging* than in conventional radiography, as there are more object parameters affecting the image and their relative contributions are very dependent on the particular imaging technique used. As in other kinds of imaging, image contrast in NMR will also depend on region size, as reflected through the modulation transfer function (MTF) characteristics.

CP—see Carr-Purcell.

CPMG—see Carr-Purcell-Meiboom-Gill.

CPU—see Computer.

Crossed-coil—*coil* pair arranged with their *magnetic fields* at right angles to each other in such a way as to minimize their mutual electromagnetic interaction.

Cryomagnet—See Superconducting magnet.

Cryostat—an apparatus for maintaining a constant low temperature (as by means of liquid helium). Requires vacuum chambers to help with thermal isolation.

CW—see Continuous wave.

DAC—see Digital to analog converter.

Data system—see Computer.

dB/dt—the rate of change of the *magnetic field* (induction) with time. Because changing magnetic fields can induce electrical fields, this is one area of potential concern for safety limits.

Demodulator—another term for *detector,* by analogy to broadcast radio receivers.

Detector—portion of the *receiver* that demodulates the *RF NMR signal* and converts it to a lower *frequency* signal. Most detectors now used are *phase* sensitive (e.g. *quadrature demodulator/detector*), and will also give phase information about the RF signal.

Diamagnetic—a substance that will slightly decrease a *magnetic field* when placed within it (its magnetization is oppositely directed to the magnetic field, i.e., with a small negative *magnetic susceptibility*).

Diffusion—the process by which molecules or other particles intermingle and migrate due to their random thermal motion. *NMR* provides a sensitive technique for measuring diffusion of some substances.

Digital to analog converter (DAC)—part of the *interface* that converts digital numbers from the *computer* into analog (ordinary) voltages or currents.

Echo—see Spin echo.

Echo planar imaging—a technique of *planar imaging* in which a complete planar image is obtained from one *selective excitation pulse*. The *FID* is observed while periodically switching the *y-gradient field* in the presence of a static *x-gradient field*. The *Fourier transform* of the resulting *spin echo* train can be used to produce an image of the excited plane.

Eddy currents—electric currents induced in a conductor by a changing *magnetic field* or by motion of the conductor through a magnetic field. One of the sources of concern about potential hazard to subjects in very high *magnetic fields* or rapidly varying *gradient* or main magnetic fields. Can be a practical problem in the *cryostat* of *superconducting magnets*.

Excitation—putting energy into the *spin* system; if a net *transverse magnetization* is produced, an *NMR signal* can be observed.

f—see Frequency.

Faraday shield—electrical conductor interposed between *transmitter and/or receiver coil* and patient to block out electric fields.

Fast Fourier transform (FFT)—an efficient computational method of performing a *Fourier transform*.

Ferromagnetic—a substance, such as iron, that has a large positive *magnetic susceptibility*.

FFT—see Fast Fourier transform.

FID—see Free induction decay.

Field gradient—see Gradient magnetic field.

Field lock—a feedback control used to maintain the static *magnetic field* at a constant strength, usually by monitoring the *resonance frequency* of a reference sample or line in the *spectrum*.

Filling factor— a measure of the geometrical relationship of the *RF coil* and the body. It affects the efficiency of irradiating the body and detecting *NMR signals,* thereby affecting the *signal-to-noise ratio* and, ultimately, image quality. Achieving a high filling factor requires fitting the coil closely to the body, thus potentially decreasing patient comfort.

Filtered back projection—mathematical technique used in *reconstruction from projections* to create images from a set of multiple *projection profiles.* It essentially involves "correcting" the projection profiles by convolving them with a suitable mathematical filter and then back projecting the filtered projections into image space. Widely used in conventional computed tomography (CT).

Flip angle—amount of rotation of the *macroscopic magnetization vector* produced by an *RF pulse,* with respect to the direction of the static *magnetic field.*

Fourier transform (FT)—a mathematical procedure to separate out the *frequency* components of a signal from its amplitudes as a function of time, or vice versa. The Fourier transform is used to generate the *spectrum* from the *FID* in *pulse NMR* techniques and is essential to most imaging techniques.

Fourier transform imaging—*NMR imaging* techniques in which at least one dimension is phase encoded by applying variable *gradient pulses* along that dimension before "reading out" the *NMR signal* with a *gradient magnetic field* perpendicular to the variable gradient. The *Fourier transform* is then used to reconstruct an image from the set of encoded NMR signals. An imaging technique of this type is *spin warp imaging.*

Free induction decay (FID)—if *transverse magnetization* of the *spins* is produced, e.g., by a *90° pulse,* a transient *NMR signal* will result that will decay toward zero with a characteristic time constant *T2* (or *T2**); this decaying signal is the FID. In practice, the first part of the FID is not observable due to residual effects of the powerful exciting *RF pulse* on the electronics of the *receiver.*

Free induction signal (FIS)—see <u>Free induction decay.</u>

Frequency (f)—the number of repetitions of a periodic process per unit time. For electromagnetic radiation, such as radio waves, the old unit, cycles per second (cps), has been replaced by the *SI* unit, *hertz,* abbreviated *Hz.* It is related to *angular frequency,* ω, by $f = \omega/2\pi$.

FT—see <u>Fourier transform.</u>

G—see Gauss.

G_x, G_y, G_z—conventional symbols for *gradient magnetic field*. Used with subscripts to denote *spatial direction* component of gradient, i.e., direction along which the field changes.

Gauss (G)—a unit of magnetic flux density in the older (CGS) system. The Earth's magnetic field is approximately one half gauss to one gauss, depending on location. The currently preferred (*SI*) unit is the *tesla* (T) (1 T = 10,000 G).

Golay coil—term commonly used for a particular kind of *gradient coil*, commonly used to create *gradient magnetic fields*, perpendicular to the main *magnetic field*.

Gradient—the amount and direction of the rate of change in space of some quantity, such as *magnetic field* strength.

Gradient coils—current carrying *coils* designed to produce a desired *gradient magnetic field* (so that the *magnetic field* will be stronger in some locations than others). Proper design of the size and configuration of the coils is necessary to produce a controlled and uniform *gradient*.

Gradient magnetic field—a *magnetic field* which changes in strength in a certain given direction. Such fields are used in *NMR imaging* with *selective excitation* to select a region for imaging and also to encode the location of *NMR signals* received from the object being imaged. Measured (e.g.) in *teslas* per meter.

Gradient pulse—briefly applied *gradient magnetic field*.

Gyromagnetic ratio (γ)—the ratio of the *magnetic moment* to the *angular momentum* of a particle. This is a constant for a given nucleus.

H_0—conventional symbol historically used for the constant *magnetic field* in an *NMR* system; it is physically more correct to use B_0. A magnet provides a field strength, H; however, at a point in an object, the *spins* experience the *magnetic induction, B*.

H_1—conventional symbol historically used for the *radiofrequency magnetic field* in an *NMR* system; it is physically more correct to use B_1. It is useful to consider it as composed of two oppositely rotating *vectors*. At the *Larmor frequency*, the vector rotating in the same direction as the *precessing spins* will interact strongly with the *spins*.

Hardware—electrical and mechanical components of *computer.*

Helmholtz coil—pair of current carrying *coils* used to create uniform *magnetic field* in the space between them.

Hertz (Hz)—the standard (*SI*) unit of *frequency*; equal to the old unit cycles per second.

Homogeneity—uniformity. In *NMR*, the homogeneity of the static *magnetic field* is an important criterion of the quality of the magnet. Homogeneity requirements for *NMR imaging* are generally lower than the homogeneity requirements for NMR spectroscopy, but for most imaging techniques must be maintained over a larger region.

Hz—see Hertz.

I—see Nuclear spin number.

Image acquisition time—time required to carry out an *NMR imaging* procedure comprising only the data acquisition time. The additional image reconstruction time will also be important to determine how quickly the image can be viewed. In comparing *sequential plane imaging* and *volume imaging* techniques, the equivalent image acquisition time per slice must be considered, as well as the actual image aquisition time.

Inductance—measure of the magnetic coupling between two current carrying loops (mutual) (reflecting their spatial relationship) or of a loop (such as a *coil*) with itself (self). One of the principal determinants of the *resonance frequency* of an *RF* circuit.

Inhomogeneity—degree of lack of *homogeneity*, for example the fractional deviation of the local *magnetic field* from the average value of the field.

Interface—set of devices that enables the interaction of the *computer* and the *spectrometer.* Particularly, this includes an *analog to digital converter* (ADC), which turns the analog voltages, such as the output of the RF *receiver,* into numbers that can be read by the *computer.* It also includes a *digital to analog converter* (DAC), which does the reverse, enabling the computer to produce control voltages.

Interpulse time—times between successive RF *pulses* used in *pulse sequences.* Particularly important are the *inversion time* (*TI*) in *inversion recovery,* and the time between a *90° pulse* and the subsequent *180° pulse* to produce a *spin echo,* which will be approximately one half the *spin echo time* (*TE*). The time between repetitions of pulse sequences is the *repetition time* (*TR*).

Inversion—a nonequilibrium state in which the *macroscopic magnetization vector* is oriented opposite to the *magnetic field*; usually produced by *adiabatic fast passage* or *180° RF pulses.*

Inversion-recovery (IR)—*pulse NMR* technique which can be incorporated into *NMR imaging,* wherein the nuclear magnetization is inverted at a time on the order of *T1* before the regular imaging pulse-gradient sequences. The resulting partial *relaxation* of the spins in the different structures being imaged can be used to produce an image that depends strongly on T1. This may bring out differences in the appearance of structures with different T1 relaxation times. Note that this does <u>not</u> directly produce an image of T1. T1 in a given region can be calculated from the change in the *NMR signal* from the region due to the inversion pulse compared to the signal with no inversion pulse or an inversion pulse with a different inversion time (TI).

Inversion time (TI)— time between *inversion* and subsequent *90° pulse* to elicit *NMR signal* in *inversion-recovery.*

Inversion transfer—see <u>Saturation transfer.</u>

IR—see <u>Inversion recovery.</u>

k—Boltzmann's constant: appears in *Boltzmann distribution.*

kHz—see <u>Kilohertz.</u>

Kilohertz (kHz)—unit of *frequency*; equal to one thousand *hertz.*

Larmor equation—states that the *frequency* of precession of the nuclear *magnetic moment* is proportional to the *magnetic field.*

$$\omega_0 = -\gamma B_0 \text{ (radians per second)}$$
$$\text{or } f_0 = -\gamma B_0 / 2\pi \text{ (hertz)}$$

where ω_0 or f_0 is the *frequency,* γ is the *gyromagnetic ratio,* and B_0 is the *magnetic induction field.* The negative sign indicates the direction of the rotation.

Larmor frequency (ω_0 or f_0)—the frequency at which magnetic resonance can be excited; given by the *Larmor equation.* By varying the *magnetic field* across the body with a *gradient magnetic field,* the corresponding variation of the Larmor frequency can be used to encode position. For protons (hydrogen nuclei), the Larmor frequency is 42.58 MH_z/tesla.

Lattice—by analogy to *NMR* in solids, the magnetic and thermal environment with which nuclei exchange energy in *longitudinal relaxation.*

Line imaging—see Sequential line imaging.

Line scanning—see Sequential line imaging.

Line width—width of line in *spectrum;* related to the reciprocal of the transverse *relaxation time* (*T2** in practical systems). Measured in units of *frequency,* generally at the half-maximum points.

LMR—see Localized magnetic resonance.

Localized magnetic resonance (LMR)—a particular technique for obtaining *NMR spectra,* for example, of phosphorus, from a limited region by creating a *sensitive volume* with *inhomogeneous* applied *gradient magnetic fields,* which may be enhanced with the use of *surface coils.*

Longitudinal magnetization (M_z)—component of the *macroscopic magnetization vector* along the static *magnetic field.* Following excitation by *RF pulse,* M_z will approach its equilibrium value M_O, with a characteristic time constant *T1.*

Longitudinal relaxation—return of *longitudinal magnetization* to its equilibrium value after *excitation;* requires exchange of energy between the *nuclear spins* and the *lattice.*

Longitudinal relaxation time—see T1.

Lorentzian line—usual shape of the lines in an *NMR spectrum,* characterized by a central peak with long tails; proportional to $1/[(1/T2)^2 + (f - f_0)^2]$, where *f* is *frequency* and f_O is the frequency of the peak (i.e., central resonance frequency).

M—conventional symbol for *macroscopic magnetization vector.*

M_{xy}—see Transverse magnetization.

M_z—see Longitudinal magnetization.

M_0—equilibrium value of the *magnetization;* directed along the direction of the static *magnetic field.* Proportional to *spin density, N.*

Macroscopic magnetic moment—see Macroscopic magnetization vector.

Macroscopic magnetization vector—net *magnetic moment* per unit volume (a *vector* quantity) of a sample in a given region, considered as the integrated effect of all the individual microscopic nuclear magnetic moments. Most *NMR* experiments actually deal with this.

Magnetic dipole—north and south magnetic poles separated by a finite distance. An electric current loop, including the effective current of a spinning nucleon or nucleus, can create an equivalent magnetic dipole.

Magnetic field (H)—the region surrounding a magnet (or current carrying conductor) is endowed with certain properties. One is that a small magnet in such a region experiences a *torque* that tends to align it in a given direction. Magnetic field is a *vector* quantity; the direction of the field is defined as the direction that the north pole of the small magnet points when in equilibrium. A magnetic field produces a magnetizing force on a body within it. Although the dangers of large magnetic fields are largely hypothetical, this is an area of potential concern for safety limits.

Formally, the forces experienced by moving charged particles, current carrying wires, and small magnets in the vicinity of a magnet are due to *magnetic induction* (B), which includes the effect of *magnetization,* while the magnetic field (H) is defined so as not to include magnetization. However, both B and H are often loosely used to denote magnetic fields.

Magnetic field gradient—see Gradient magnetic field.

Magnetic induction (B)—also called magnetic flux density. The net magnetic effect from an externally applied *magnetic field* and the resulting *magnetization.* B is proportional to H ($B = \mu H$), with the *SI* unit being the *tesla.*

Magnetic moment—a measure of the net magnetic properties of an object or particle. A nucleus with an intrinsic *spin* will have an associated *magnetic dipole* moment, so that it will interact with a *magnetic field* (as if it were a tiny bar magnet).

Magnetic resonance—see Nuclear magnetic resonance (NMR). Another magnetic resonance phenomenon is electron spin resonance (ESR).

Magnetic susceptibility (χ)—measure of the ability of a substance to become magnetized.

Magnetization (see also Macroscopic magnetization vector)—the magnetic polarization of a material produced by a *magnetic field* (magnetic moment per unit volume).

Magnetogyric ratio—see Gyromagnetic ratio.

Maxwell coil—a particular kind of *gradient coil*, commonly used to create *gradient magnetic fields* along the direction of the main *magnetic field*.

Megahertz (MHz)—unit of *frequency*, equal to one million *hertz*.

Meiboom-Gill sequence—see Carr-Purcell-Meiboom-Gill sequence.

MHz—see Megahertz.

Multiple line-scan imaging (MLSI)—variation of *sequential line imaging* techniques that can be used if *selective excitation* methods that do not affect adjacent lines are employed. Adjacent lines are imaged while waiting for *relaxation* of the first line toward equilibrium, which may result in decreased *imaging time*. A different type of MLSI uses simultaneous excitation of two or more lines with different phase encoding followed by suitable decoding.

Multiple plane imaging—variation of *sequential plane imaging* techniques that can be used with *selective excitation* techniques that do not affect adjacent planes. Adjacent planes are imaged while waiting for relaxation of the first plane toward equilibrium, resulting in decreased *imaging time*.

Multiple sensitive point—*sequential line imaging* technique utilizing two orthogonal oscillating *magnetic field gradients,* an *SFP* pulse sequence, and signal averaging to isolate the *NMR spectrometer* sensitivity to a desired line in the body.

N (H)—see Spin density.

NMR—see Nuclear magnetic resonance.

NMR imaging (see also Zeugmatography)—creation of images of objects such as the body by use of the *nuclear magnetic resonance* phenomenon. The immediate practical application involves imaging the distribution of hydrogen nuclei (protons) in the body. The image brightness in a given region is usually dependent jointly on the *spin density* and the *relaxation times,* with their relative importance determined by the particular imaging technique employed. Image brightness is also affected by motion such as blood flow.

NMR signal—electromagnetic signal in the *radiofrequency* range produced by the *precession* of the *transverse magnetization* of the *spins*. The rotation of the transverse magnetization induces a voltage in a *coil,* which is amplified and demodulated by the *receiver*; the signal may refer only to this induced voltage.

Nuclear magnetic resonance (NMR)—the absorption or emission of electromagnetic energy by nuclei in a static *magnetic field,* after *excitation* by a suitable RF magnetic field. The peak *resonance frequency* is proportional to the magnetic field, and is given by the *Larmor equation.* Only nuclei with a non-zero *spin* exhibit NMR.

Nuclear signal—see NMR signal.

Nuclear spin (see also Spin)—an intrinsic property of certain nuclei that gives them an associated characteristic *angular momentum* and *magnetic moment.*

Nuclear spin quantum number (I)—property of all nuclei related to the largest measurable component of the nuclear *angular momentum.* Non zero values of nuclear angular momentum are quantized (fixed) as integral or half-integral multiples of $(h/2\pi)$, where h is Planck's constant. The number of possible energy states for a given nucleus in a fixed *magnetic field* is equal to $2I + 1$.

Nucleon—generic term for a neutron or proton.

Nutation—a displacement of the axis of a spinning body away from the simple coneshaped figure which would be traced by the axis during *precession.* In the *rotating frame of reference,* the nutation caused by an *RF pulse* appears as a simple precession, although the motion is more complex in the stationary frame of reference.

Orientation—a suggested standard orientation for the presentation of *NMR* images is: 1) transverse: patient's right on the left side of the image, anterior or ventral on top, 2) coronal: patient's right to left side of image, superior or head to the top, 3) sagittal: patient's head to the top, anterior to the left side of image. R, L, S and A should be shown on the screen, as appropriate. In displaying sagittal images, it is helpful to indicate whether a slice is to the left or right of the midline.

Paramagnetic—a substance with a small but positive *magnetic susceptibity* (magnetizability). The addition of a small amount of paramagnetic substance may greatly reduce the *relaxation times* of water. Typical paramagnetic substances usually possess an unpaired electron and include atoms or ions of transition elements, rare earth elements, some metals, and some molecules including molecular oxygen and free radicals. Paramagnetic substances are considered promising for use as contrast agents in *NMR imaging.*

Partial saturation (PS)—*excitation technique* applying repeated *RF pulses* in times on the order of or shorter than *T1.* In *NMR imaging* systems, although it results in decreased signal amplitude, there is the possibility of generating images with increased *contrast* between regions with different *relaxation times.* It does not directly produce images of T1. The change in NMR signal from a region resulting from a change in the *interpulse time, TR,* can be used to calculate T1 for the region. Although partial saturation is also commonly referred to as *saturation recovery,* that term should properly be reserved for the particular case of partial saturation in which recovery after each *excitation* effectively takes place from true *saturation.*

Permanent magnet—a magnet whose *magnetic field* originates from permanently magnetized material.

Permeability (μ)—tendency of a substance to concentrate *magnetic field,* $\mu = B/H$.

Phantom—an artificial object of known dimensions and properties used to test aspects of an imaging machine.

Phase—in a periodic function (such as rotational or sinusoidal motion), the position relative to a particular part of the cycle.

Phase sensitive detector—see Demodulator.

Pixel—acronym for a picture element; the smallest discrete part of a digital image display.

Planar spin imaging—one particular technique of *planar imaging* that creates an *NMR image* of a plane from one excitation sequence by selectively exciting a grid of points within the plane and then applying a *gradient magnetic field* so that each point has a different *Larmor frequency. Fourier transformation* of the *FID* can then be used to separate the signals from each selected point and create the image.

Planar imaging--imaging technqiue in which image of a plane is built up from signals received from the whole plane. See also Sequential plane imaging.

Point imaging—see Sequential point imaging.

Point scanning—see Sequential point imaging.

Precession—comparatively slow gyration of the axis of a spinning body so as to trace out a cone; caused by the application of a *torque* tending to change the direction of the rotation axis, and continuously directed at right angles to the plane of the torque. The *magnetic moment* of a nucleus with *spin* will experience such a torque when inclined at an angle to the *magnetic field,* resulting in precession at the *Larmor frequency.* A familiar example is the effect of gravity on the motion of a spinning top or gyroscope.

Precessional frequency—see Larmor frequency.

Probe—the portion of an *NMR spectrometer* comprising the sample container and the *RF* coils, with some associated electronics. The RF coils may consist of separate *receiver* and *transmitter* coils in a *crossed-coil* configuration, or, alternatively, a single coil to perform both functions.

Program—see Software.

Progressive saturation—see Saturation recovery.

Projection profile—*spectrum* of *NMR signal* whose *frequency* components are broadened by a *gradient magnetic field.* In the simplest case (negligible *line width,* no *relaxation* effects, and no effects of prior gradients), it corresponds to a one-dimensional projection of the *spin density* along the direction of the gradient; in this form it is used in *reconstruction from projections imaging.*

PS—see Partial saturation.

Pulse, 90° ($\pi/2$ **pulse**)—*RF pulse* designed to rotate the *macroscopic magnetization vector* 90° in space as referred to the *rotating frame of reference,* usually about an axis at right angles to the main *magnetic field.* If the *spins* are initially aligned with the magnetic field, this pulse will produce *transverse magnetization* and an *FID.*

Pulse, 180° (π **pulse**)—*RF pulse* designed to rotate the *macroscopic magnetization vector* 180° in space as referred to the *rotating frame of reference,* usually about an axis at right angles to the main *magnetic field.* If the *spins* are initially aligned with the magnetic field, this pulse will produce *inversion.*

Pulse, RF—see RF pulse.

Pulse length (width)—time duration of a *pulse.* For an *RF pulse* near the *Larmor frequency,* the longer the pulse length, the greater the angle of rotation of the *macroscopic magnetization vector* will be (greater than 180° can bring it back toward its original orientation).

Pulse NMR—*NMR* techniques that use *RF pulses* and *Fourier transformation* of the *NMR signal*; have largely replaced the older *continuous wave* techniques.

Pulse programmer—part of the *spectrometer* or *interface* that controls the timing, duration, and amplitude of the *pulses* (*RF* or *gradient*).

Pulse sequences--set of *RF* (and/or *gradient*) *magnetic field pulses* and time spacings between these pulses; used in conjunction with gradient magnetic fields and *NMR signal* reception to produce *NMR* images. See also Interpulse times.

Pulsed gradients—see Gradient pulse.

Q—see Quality factor.

Quadrature detector—a *phase* sensitive *detector* or *demodulator* that detects the components of the signal in phase with a reference oscillator and 90° out of phase with the reference oscillator.

Quality factor (Q)—applies to any electrical circuit component; most often the *coil* Q is limiting. Inversely related to the fraction of the energy in an oscillating system lost in one oscillation cycle. Q is inversely related to the range of *frequency* over which the system will exhibit *resonance*. It affects the *signal-to-noise ratio,* because the detected signal increases proportionally to Q while the noise is proportional to the square root of Q. The Q of a coil will depend on whether it is unloaded (no patient) or loaded (patient).

Quenching—loss of superconductivity of the current carrying coil that may occur unexpectedly in a *superconducting magnet.* As the magnet becomes resistive, heat will be released that can result in rapid evaporation of liquid helium in the *cryostat.* This may present a hazard if not properly planned for.

Radian—dimensionless unit of angular measure; $360° = 2\pi$ radians.

Radiofrequency (RF)—wave *frequency* intermediate between auditory and infra red. The RF used in *NMR* studies is commonly in the *megahertz* (MHz) range. The principal effect of RF *magnetic fields* on the body is power deposition in the form of heating, mainly at the surface; this is a principal area of concern for safety limits.

Readout delay—see TE.

Receiver—portion of the *NMR* apparatus that detects and amplifies *RF* signals picked up by the receiving *coil*. Includes a preamplifier, amplifier, and *demodulator.*

Receiver coil—*coil* of the *RF receiver*; "picks up" the *NMR signal.*

Reconstruction from projections imaging—*NMR imaging* technique in which a set of *projection profiles* of the body is obtained by observing *NMR signals* in the presence of a suitable corresponding set of *gradient magnetic fields*. Images can then be reconstructed using techniques analogous to those used in conventional computed tomography (CT), such as *filtered back projection*. It can be used for *volume imaging* or, with plane selection techniques, for *sequential plane imaging.*

Refocusing—see Spin echo.

Relaxation rates—reciprocals of the *relaxation times.*

Relaxation times—after *excitation,* the *spins* will tend to return to their equilibrium distribution, in which there is no *transverse magnetization* and the *longitudinal magnetization* is at its maximum value and oriented in the direction of the static *magnetic field*. It is observed that in the absence of applied RF, the transverse magnetization decays toward zero with a characteristic time constant $T2$, and the longitudinal magnetization returns toward the equilibrium value M_0 with a characteristic time constant $T1$.

Repeated FID—a form of *NMR imaging* in which repeated *90° pulses* are applied. Results in *partial saturation* if interpulse times are of the order of or less than $T1$. Strictly speaking, applies only if *NMR* signal is detected as an *FID.*

Repetition time—see TR.

Rephasing gradient—*gradient magnetic field* applied for a brief period after a *selective excitation* pulse, in the opposite direction to the *gradient* used for the selective excitation. The result of the gradient reversal is a rephasing of the *spins* (which will have gotten out of phase with each other along the direction of the selection gradient), forming an *echo* by "*time reversal,*" and improving the sensitivity of imaging after the selective excitation process.

Resistive magnet—a magnet whose *magnetic field* originates from current flowing through an ordinary (nonsuperconducting) conductor.

Resolution, spatial—although generally referring to the ability of the imaging process to distinguish adjacent structures in the object (an important measure of image quality), the specific criterion of resolution to be used depends on the type of test used (e.g. bar pattern or contrast-detail *phantom*). As the ability to separate or detect objects depends on their *contrast*, and the different *NMR* parameters of objects will affect image contrast differently for different imaging techniques, care must be taken in comparing the results of resolution *phantom* tests of different machines and no single simple measure of resolution can be specified.

Resonance—a large amplitude vibration in a mechanical or electrical system caused by a relatively small periodic stimulus with a *frequency* at or close to a natural frequency of the system; in *NMR* apparatus, resonance can refer to the NMR itself or to the tuning of the *RF* circuitry.

Resonant frequency—frequency at which *resonance* phenomenon occurs; given by the *Larmor equation* for *NMR*; determined by *inductance* and capacitance for *RF* circuits.

RF—see Radiofrequency.

RF coil—used for transmitting *RF pulses* and/or receiving *NMR signals*. Most commonly used in *saddle coil* or *solenoid* configurations for *NMR imaging*.

RF pulse—brief burst of *RF magnetic field* delivered to object by *RF transmitter.* For *RF frequency* near the *Larmor frequency,* it will result in rotation of the *macroscopic magnetization vector* in the *rotating frame of reference* (or a more complicated *nutational* motion in the stationary frame of reference). The amount of rotation will depend on the strength and duration of the RF pulse; commonly used examples are *90° ($\pi/2$)* and *180° (π) pulses.*

Rotating frame of reference—a frame of reference (with corresponding coordinate systems) that is rotating about the axis of the static *magnetic field B_0* (with respect to a stationary ("laboratory") frame of reference) at a *frequency* equal to that of the applied *RF* magnetic field, B_1. Although B_1 is a rotating *vector,* it appears stationary in the rotating frame, leading to simpler mathematical formulations.

Rotating frame zeugmatography—technique of *NMR imaging* that uses a *gradient* of the *RF excitation* field (to give a corresponding variation of the *flip angle* along the gradient as a means of encoding the spatial location of *spins* in the direction of the RF field gradient) in conjunction with a static *gradient magnetic field* (to give spatial encoding in an orthogonal direction). It can be considered to be a form of *Fourier transform imaging.*

Saddle coil—*RF coil* configuration design commonly used when the static *magnetic field* is coaxial with the axis of the coil along the long axis of the body (e.g. *superconducting magnets* and most *resistive magnets*) as opposed to solenoid or surface coil.

Saturation—a nonequilibrium state in *NMR*, in which equal numbers of *spins* are aligned against and with the *magnetic field*, so that there is no net *magnetization*. Can be produced by repeatedly supplying *RF* pulses at the *Larmor frequency* with interpulse times short compared to *T1*.

Saturation recovery (SR)—particular type of *partial saturation pulse sequence* in which the preceding pulses leave the *spins* in a state of *saturation*, so that recovery at the time of the next pulse has taken place from an initial condition of no magnetization.

Saturation transfer (or Inversion transfer)—nuclei can retain their magnetic orientation through a chemical reaction. Thus, if *RF* radiation is supplied to the *spins* at a *frequency* corresponding to the *chemical shift* of the nuclei in one chemical state so as to produce *saturation* or *inversion*, and chemical reactions transform the nuclei into another chemical state with a different chemical shift in a time short compared to the *relaxation time*, the *NMR spectrum* may show the effects of the saturation or inversion on the corresponding, unirradiated, line in the spectrum. This technique can be used to study reaction kinetics of suitable molecules.

SE—see <u>Spin echo.</u>

Selective excitation—controlling the *frequency spectrum* of an irradiating *RF pulse* (via *tailoring*) while imposing a *gradient magnetic field* on *spins*, such that only a desired region will have a suitable *resonant frequency* to be excited. Originally used to excite all but a desired region; now more commonly used to select only a desired region, such as a plane, for excitation.

Selective irradiation—see <u>Selective excitation.</u>

Sensitive plane—technique of selecting a plane for *sequential plane imaging* by using an oscillating *gradient magnetic field* and filtering out the corresponding time-dependent part of the *NMR signal*. The *gradient* used is at right angles to the desired plane and the magnitude of the oscillating gradient magnetic field is equal to zero only in the desired plane.

Sensitive point—technique of selecting out a point for *sequential point imaging* by applying three orthogonal oscillating *gradient magnetic fields* such that the local *magnetic field* is time dependent everywhere except at the desired point, and then filtering out the corresponding time dependent portion of the *NMR signal*.

Sensitive volume—region of the object from which *NMR signal* will preferentially be acquired because of strong *magnetic field inhomogeneity* elsewhere. Effect can be enhanced by use of a shaped *RF* field that is strongest in the sensitive region.

Sequence time—see TR.

Sequential line imaging (Line scanning, Line imaging)—*NMR imaging* techniques in which the image is built up from successive lines through the object. In various schemes, the lines are isolated by oscillating *gradient magnetic fields* or *selective excitation,* and then the *NMR signals* from the selected line are encoded for position by detecting the *FID* or *spin echo* in the presence of a gradient magnetic field along the line; the *Fourier transform* of the detected signal then yields the distribution of emitted NMR signal along the line.

Sequential plane imaging (Plane imaging)—*NMR imaging* technique in which the image of an object is built up from successive planes in the object. In various schemes, the planes are selected by oscillating *gradient magnetic fields* or *selective excitation.*

Sequential point imaging (Point scanning)—*NMR imaging* techniques in which the image is built from successive point positions in the object. In various schemes, the points are isolated by oscillating *gradient magnetic fields (sensitive point)* or shaped *magnetic fields.*

SFP—see Steady state free precession.

Shim coils—*coils* carrying a relatively small current that are used to provide auxiliary *magnetic fields* in order to compensate for *inhomogeneities* in the main magnetic field of an *NMR* system.

Shimming—correction of *inhomogeneity* of the *magnetic field* produced by the main magnet of an *NMR* system due to imperfections in the magnet or to the presence of external *ferromagnetic* objects. May involve changing the configuration of the magnet or the addition of *shim coils* or small pieces of steel.

SI (International System of Units)—the preferred international standard system of physical units and measures.

Signal-to-noise ratio (SNR or S/N)—used to describe the relative contributions to a detected signal of the true signal and random superimposed signals ("noise"). One common method to improve (increase) the SNR is to average several measurements of the signal on the expectation that random contributions will tend to cancel out. The SNR can also be improved by sampling larger volumes (with a corresponding loss of spatial *resolution*) or, within limits, by increasing the strength of the *magnetic field* used. S/N will depend on the electrical properties of the sample or patient being studied.

Simultaneous volume imaging—see Volume imaging.

Skin depth—time dependent electromagnetic fields are significantly attenuated by conducting media (including the human body); the skin depth gives a measure of the average depth of penetration of the *RF* field. It may be a limiting factor in *NMR imaging* at very high frequencies (high *magnetic fields*). The skin depth also affects the *Q* of the *coils*.

S/N—see Signal-to-noise ratio.

SNR—see Signal-to-noise ratio.

Software—the set of instructions, or programs, that controls the activities of the *computer*. Programs may be written in machine language (sequences of numbers directly interpretable by the computer), assembly language, or higher level languages such as Fortran or Basic. The software includes overall supervising "executive" programs, data acquisition programs, data processing programs (including image reconstruction), and display programs.

Solenoid coil—a coil of wire wound in the form of a long cylinder. When a current is passed through the coil, the *magnetic field* within the coil is relatively uniform. Solenoid *RF coils* are commonly used when the static magnetic field is perpendicular to the long axis of the body.

Spectrometer—the portions of the *NMR* apparatus that actually produce the NMR phenomenon and acquire the signals, including the magnet, the *probe,* the *RF* circuitry, etc. The spectrometer is controlled by the *computer* via the *interface* under the direction of the *software*.

Spectrum—an array of the frequency components of the *NMR signal* according to *frequency.* Nuclei with different *resonant frequencies* will show up as peaks at different corresponding frequencies in the spectrum, or "lines."

Spin—the intrinsic *angular momentum* of an elementary particle, or system of particles such as a nucleus, that is also responsible for the *magnetic moment;* or, a particle or nucleus possessing such a spin. The spins of nuclei have characteristic fixed values. Pairs of neutrons and protons align to cancel out their spins, so that nuclei with an odd number of neutrons and/or protons will have a net nonzero rotational component characterized by an integer or half integer quantum *"nuclear spin number"* (I).

Spin density (N)—the density of resonating *spins* in a given region; one of the principal determinants of the strength of the *NMR signal* from the region. The SI units would be moles/m^3. For water, there are about 1.1×10^5 moles of hydrogen per m^3, or .11 moles of hydrogen/cm^3. True spin density is <u>not</u> imaged directly, but must be calculated from signals received with different *interpulse times*.

Spin echo—reappearance of an *NMR signal* after the *FID* has died away, as a result of the effective reversal of the dephasing of the *spins* ("refocusing") by such techniques as reversal of a *gradient magnetic field* (often referred to as a form of *"time reversal"*), or by specific *RF pulse* sequences such as the *Carr-Purcell sequence* (applied in a time shorter than or on the order of *T2*). Multiple spin echoes or a series of spin echoes at different times can be used to determine T2 without contamination by effects of the *inhomogeneity* of the *magnetic field.*

Spin-echo imaging—any of many *NMR imaging* techniques in which the *spin echo NMR signal* rather than the *FID* is used. Can be used to create images that depend strongly on *T2*. Note that spin echoes do <u>not</u> directly produce an image of T2.

Spin-lattice relaxation time—see <u>T1</u>.

Spin number, nuclear—see <u>Nuclear spin number</u>.

Spin—Spin relaxation time—see <u>T2</u>.

Spin tagging—nuclei will retain their magnetic orientation for a time on the order of *T1* even in the presence of motion. Thus, if the nuclei in a given region have their spin orientation changed, the altered spins will serve as a "tag" to trace the motion of any fluid that may have been in the tagged region for a time on the order of T1.

Spin warp imaging—a form of *Fourier transform imaging* in which *phase* encoding *gradient pulses* are applied for a constant duration but with varying amplitude. This is distinct from the original *FT* imaging methods in which phase encoding is performed by applying gradient pulses of constant amplitude but varying duration. The spin warp method, as other Fourier imaging techniques, is relatively tolerant of nonuniformities (*inhomogeneities*) in the static or *gradient magnetic fields.*

SR—see <u>Saturation recovery</u>.

SSFP—see <u>Steady state free precession</u>.

Steady state free precession (SFP or SSFP)—method of *NMR excitation* in which strings of *RF pulses* are applied rapidly and repeatedly with interpulse intervals short compared to both *T1* and *T2*. Alternating the phases of the RF pulses by 180° can be useful in obtaining maximal signal strength.

Superconducting magnet—a magnet whose *magnetic field* originates from current flowing through a *superconductor.* Such a magnet must be enclosed in a *cryostat.*

Superconductor—a substance whose electrical resistance essentially disappears at temperatures near absolute zero. A commonly used superconductor in *NMR imaging* system magnets is niobium-titanium, embedded in a copper matrix to help protect the superconductor from *quenching.*

Surface coil NMR—a simple flat *RF receiver coil* placed over a region of interest will have an effective selectivity for a volume approximately subtended by the coil circumference and one radius deep from the coil center. Such a coil can be used for simple localization of sites for measurement of *chemical shift spectra,* especially of phosphorus, and blood flow studies. Some additional spatial selectivity can be achieved with *gradient magnetic fields.*

Susceptibility—see Magnetic susceptibility.

T—see Tesla.

T1 ("**T-one**")—spin-lattice or longitudinal *relaxation time;* the characteristic time constant for *spins* to tend to align themselves with the external *magnetic field.* Starting from zero *magnetization* in the z direction, the z magnetization will grow to 63% of its final maximum value in a time T1.

T2 ("**T-two**")—spin-spin or transverse *relaxation time;* the characteristic time constant for loss of *phase coherence* among *spins* oriented at an angle to the static *magnetic field,* due to interactions between the spins, with resulting loss of *transverse magnetization* and *NMR signal.* Starting from a non zero value of the *magnetization* in the xy plane, the xy magnetization will decay so that it loses 63% of its initial value in a time T2.

T2* ("**T-two-star**")—the characteristic time constant for loss of *phase coherence* among *spins* oriented at an angle to the static *magnetic field* due to a combination of magnetic field *inhomogeneities,* ΔB, and spin-spin transverse relaxation with resultant more rapid loss in *transverse magnetization* and *NMR signal.* NMR signal can still be recovered as a *spin echo* in times less than or on the order of *T2.* $1/T2^* = 1/T2 + \Delta\omega/2$; $\Delta\omega = \gamma\Delta B$.

Tailored excitation—see Selective excitation.

Tailored pulse—shaped pulse whose magnitude is varied with time in a predetermined manner. Affects the *frequency* components of an *RF pulse* in a manner determined by the *Fourier transform* of the pulse.

TE—*echo time.* Time between middle of *90° pulse* and middle of *spin echo* production. For multiple echoes, use TE1, TE2. . . .

Tesla (T)—the preferred (*SI*) unit of magnetic flux density. One tesla is equal to 10,000 *gauss,* the older (CGS) unit.

Thermal equilibrium—a state in which all parts of a system are at the same effective temperature, in particular where the relative alignment of the *spins* with the *magnetic field* is determined solely by the thermal energy of the system (in which case the relative numbers of spins with different alignments will be given by the *Boltzmann distribution).*

TI—*inversion* time. Time after middle of inverting *RF pulse* to middle of *90° pulse* to detect amount of *longitudinal magnetization.*

Time reversal—technique of producing a *spin echo* by subjecting *excited* spins to a *gradient magnetic field,* and then reversing the direction of the gradient field. All methods of spin echo production can be viewed as effective time reversal.

Torque—the effectiveness of a force in setting a body into rotation. It is a *vector* quantity given by the vector product of the force and the position vector where the force is applied; for a rotating body, the torque is the product of the moment of inertia and the resulting angular acceleration.

TR—repetition time. The period of time between the beginning of a *pulse sequence* and the beginning of the succeeding (essentially identical) pulse sequence.

Transmitter—portion of the *NMR* apparatus that produces *RF* current and delivers it to the transmitting *coil.*

Transmitter coil—*coil* of the *RF transmitter.*

Transverse magnetization (M_{xy})—component of the *macroscopic magnetization vector* at right angles to the static *magnetic field (B_o).* *Precession* of the transverse magnetization at the *Larmor frequency* is responsible for the detectable *NMR signal.* In the absence of externally applied *RF* energy, the transverse magnetization will decay to zero with a characteristic time constant of *T2* or *T2*.*

Transverse relaxation time—see T2.

Two-dimensional Fourier transform imaging (2DFT)—a form of *sequential plane imaging* using *Fourier transform imaging.*

Tuning—process of adjusting the *resonant frequency,* e.g., of the *RF* circuit, to a desired value, e.g., the *Larmor frequency.* More generally, the process of adjusting the components of the *spectrometer* for optimal *NMR signal* strength.

Tunnel—opening into *NMR imaging* machine to place patient into imaging region.

Vector—a quantity having both magnitude and direction, frequently represented by an arrow whose length is proportional to the magnitude and with an arrowhead at one end to indicate the direction.

Volume imaging—imaging techniques in which *NMR signals* are gathered from the whole object volume to be imaged at once, with appropriate encoding *pulse/gradient* sequences to encode positions of the *spins*. Many *sequential plane imaging* techniques can be generalized to volume imaging, at least in principle. Advantages include potential improvement in *signal-to-noise ratio* by including signal from the whole volume at once; disadvantages include a bigger computational task for image reconstruction and longer *image acquisition times* (although the entire volume can be imaged from the one set of data). Also called simultaneous volume imaging.

Voxel—volume element; the element of 3-D space corresponding to a *pixel,* for a given slice thickness.

x—dimension in the stationary (laboratory) frame of reference in the plane orthogonal (at right angles) to the direction of the static *magnetic field* (B_O), z, and orthogonal to *y*, the other dimension in this plane.

x^1—dimension in the *rotating frame of reference* in the plane at right angles to the direction of the static *magnetic field* (B_O), z; defined to be in the direction of the magnetic *vector* of the *RF* field (B_1).

y—dimension in the stationary (laboratory) frame of reference in the plane orthogonal to the direction of the static *magnetic field* (B_O and H_O), z, and orthogonal to *x*, the other dimension in this plane.

y^1—dimension in the *rotating frame of reference* in the plane orthogonal (at right angles) to the direction of the static *magnetic field* (B_O and H_O), z, and orthogonal to the other dimension in this plane, x^1.

z—dimension in the direction of the static *magnetic field* (B_O and H_O), in both the stationary and *rotating frames of reference.*

Zeugmatography—term for *NMR imaging* coined from Greek roots suggesting the role of the *gradient magnetic field* in joining the *RF* magnetic field to a desired local spatial region through *nuclear magnetic resonance.*

2DFT—see Two-dimensional Fourier transform.

γ—see Gyromagnetic ratio.

δ—see Chemical shift.

μ—see Permeability.

ς—often used to denote different time delays between *RF pulses.* See Interpulse times.

χ—see Magnetic susceptibility.

ω—see Angular frequency.

ω_0—see Larmor frequency.

Index

Abdominal MR imaging, 131, 134-36
Abscess formation, 97
Absorption peaks, 160
Acoustic neuroma, 102
Acute myocardial infarction, 125
Adenosine diphosphate, 164
Adenosine triphosphate, 164
Alcoholic cirrhosis, 139
Ambient conditions, 62
Analog-digital convertors, 55
Aortic aneurysms, 126
Aortic atherosclerosis, 128
Aortic dissection, 129
Aperture, 52
Arnold-Chiari malformations, 103
Astrocytoma, 89
  (*see also* Low grade astrocytoma)
Atherosclerotic plaques, 127
Axial magnetic field, 52

Basal metabolic rate, 45
Basilar invagination, 103
Bead-chain effect, 46
Biopotentials, 44
Bladder carcinoma, 152
Bloch, F.
  Nobel prize, 3
Blood flow, 25
Boil-off gases, 62
Bone, 98
Bounce point, 29
Brain, 170, 173
Brain stem infarction, 100
Brain tumors, 84

Breast imaging, 131
Bronchogenic carcinoma, 118

^{13}C enriched compounds, 163
Carbon-13, 163-64
Cardiac motion, 119
Cardiac muscle, 168-70
Cardiac pacemakers, 46, 59
Cardiovascular studies, 119, 121, 123-29
Carr-Purcell sequence, 31
Carr-Purcell-Meiboom-Gill sequence, 32
Central nervous system, 75-76
  normal anatomy, 77
Cerebellar tumor, 98
Cervicomedullary syrinx, 105
Cervix
  (*see* Metastic carcinoma of the cervix
Chemical shift imaging, 173-74
Chemical shifts, 160
Chiari malformations, 102-103
Cholecystitis, 140
Chromophobe adenoma, 92
Clinical limitations, 182
Colon carcinoma, 136
Computer software, 181
Cone of precession, 16
Congenital heart disease, 119, 125
Contrast agents, 9
Correlation time, 66
Cortical infarction, 82
Craniopharyngioma, 88

211